Yoga, Tantra and Meditation
in Daily Life

Swami Janakananda Saraswati (The Source of Bliss)

New translation by Kellie Williams and Robyn Taylor

New expanded and revised edition

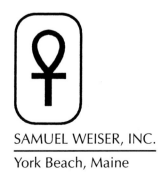

SAMUEL WEISER, INC.

York Beach, Maine

Contents

To
my Guru Swami Satyananda Saraswati,
who showed me the way to the insight
on which this book is based.

To
Swami Nityabodhananda Saraswati,
Peo, Swami Chinmudra Saraswati,
Ananda Murti, Knud Omø, Mogens
Barslund, Hari Prem, Franz Jervidalo,
Robert Nilsson, Joachim Rodenbeck,
Sita and the people in our Yoga and
Meditation Workshop, who helped with
the birth of the book and to those who
use these methods.

The symbols used in the book
communicate in their own way and
therefore have no captions.

The symbols of chapter 4 were designed
by Knud Hvidberg, Denmark. Pictures: p.
13 by Knud Hvidberg; p. 80 from a print
by Leif Madsen, Denmark; pp. 14, 15, 16,
21, 87 Ajit Mookerjee Tantra Museum,
New Delhi; p. 17 Tomas Pedersen & Stig
Andersen; p. 22 Iskcon Press, Boston; p.
23 Lars Bengtsson, Sweden; p. 24 Swami
Satyananda, India; p. 88 Siva & Parvati,
Danish National Museum; p. 99 by Bjarke,
Norway; p.100 by Christian Paaske, Norway;
p.101 by Kjeld Jensen, Denmark; pp.102,
107, 109, 110, 112, 113, 115 by Ronald
Nameth in Energy Art of Television;
p. 117 by Ellen Jensen, Denmark;
pp 5, 119 by John Cole, New York.

Photographer: Chris Stuhr, Denmark.
Layout by Swami Janakananda.

Revised American edition published
in 1992 by
Samuel Weiser, Inc.
Box 612, York Beach, ME 03910
© 1975, 1991 Swami Janakananda
Second printing, 1993
New English translation © 1991 Bindu,
Scandinavian Yoga and Meditation School

**Library of Congress Cataloging-in-Publication
Data**

Janakananda Saraswati, Swami, 1939–
    [Yoga, tantra, och meditation i min
      vardag, English]
    Yoga, tantra, and meditation in daily life
/ Swami Janakananda Saraswati: new
translation by Kellie Williams and Robyn
Taylor.——
    New, expanded, and rev. ed.
      p.   cm.
    Translation of: Yoga, tantra, och
    meditation i min vardag.
    1. Yoga.   I. Williams, Kellie.   II.
    Taylor, Robyn.   III. Title.
    B132.Y6J3513   1991
    181'.45—dc20   92–15860
                                          CIP
ISBN 0-87728-768-6

Photographs © 1975, 1981, 1986 Chris Stuhr

Printed in the United Kingdom

Part One

Introduction and Background

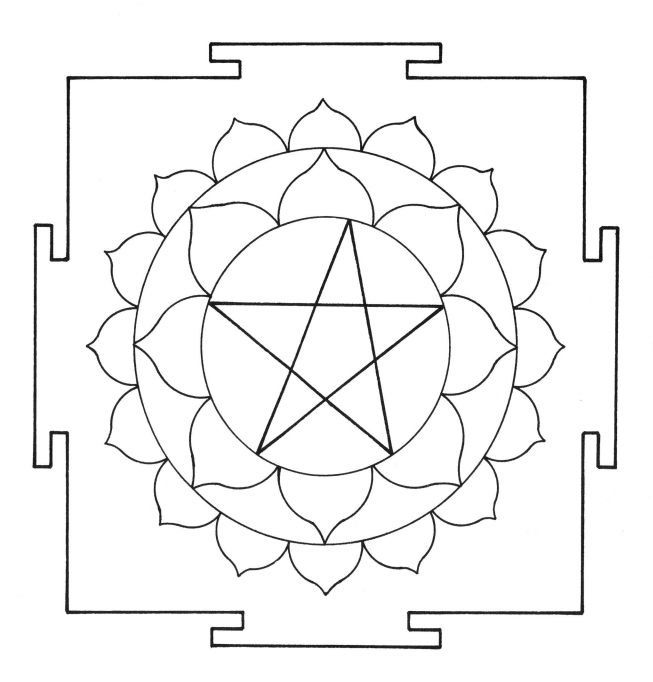

Chapter 1

Although you can follow up the practice with instructions and guidance from books, thus gaining inspiration from the experience of others, it is not enough to know about yoga just in theory.

Meditation and yoga is something that you **do**.
What use is there just talking about something you have read?
Experience you get from practice.

Only by using the various exercises and meditations will you feel an effect. And that will give you insight and inspire you to continue.
　Many of us think that yoga means we must stop living the way we do: change eating habits, stop smoking, drinking wine and, last but not least, stop having a natural sex life.
　Tantric yoga says go on living your life as you usually do. Just add another habit - yoga.

Through yoga, consciousness is expanded in a harmonic and natural way. When the body becomes strong and supple and the mind calm, you can see your life patterns, gain perspective and above all accept what you see. You become conscious.
　In this acceptance you find a peace, a foundation for self-reliance and inner contentment: a state that is not based upon something being forced on you, or upon indifference or a fearful attitude about what is allowed and what is forbidden. It is an awake, participating attitude towards whatever you meet in the extremes of life.

You do not remake yourself, you grow and become fit for life.

Yoga...

Yoga is an old Sanskrit word meaning union or **oneness**. A whole person at one with himself or herself, as opposed to an inwardly divided person.
When we wish to learn about yoga, we often think we have to sit down and learn many new terms and a philosophy. Words and philosophy gained through reading are only second-hand knowledge - which has nothing to do with yoga itself.
　Yoga is basically a tangible and practical system to help you develop as a human being.

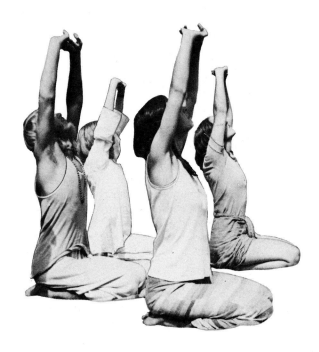

Chapter 2

Why Yoga and Meditation?

Yoga and authorities

You could spend a lifetime reading books; a lot of time is spent dreaming, philosophizing and judging. Reading about life is like giving one's beloved a novel about love - living it is something else.

Still, guidance is necessary. How does one find one's way?

The greater part of yogic literature written in recent centuries has been strongly influenced by thoughts that also dominated other parts of society, especially from the Victorian era and all that it involved.

Many yoga books unfortunately mirrored a fear of confronting life and an ignorance of what people, even today, can understand and use, and what they need. Life often became wrapped up in rules and prejudices so that a few people, who were incapable of letting go of their own fears, could maintain religious power in a rigid caste and social system. Often a truly profound practical experience of yoga and meditation was lacking.

It is no good passing on this knowledge of yoga without having digested it thoroughly. Today, however, we see independent points of view that are beginning to loosen the narrow attitudes from the past.

Yoga and meditation were not originally part of any religious system. Their objective is broader: not to bind people in ignorance and prejudice but rather to transform and develop human consciousness. In this way free and independent individuals are created, who make their own experiences, fulfil their potential, each living in a personal and truly social way.

We don't need books that talk **about** yoga and meditation. What we want is **practical** guidance and an introduction to methods and techniques.

Yoga and meditation must be a part of your daily life for some months before you can really say anything about it - even though many will feel a beneficial effect right away.

And as for your philosophy of life and your various opinions, well, that's up to you.

The common inheritance

In India, yoga has been preserved in the Tantric tradition, but meditation and yoga exercises are not exclusively Indian. We find knowledge of meditation and similar methods in such separate civilizations as those of the American Indians, the old Nordic cultures, in ancient Egypt, Babylon and Rome, in Sufism (a living Arabic tradition), in China and of course in India.

Pythagoras had a school which taught meditation amidst other studies, and the Roman emperor Marcus Aurelius wrote a book on the subject.

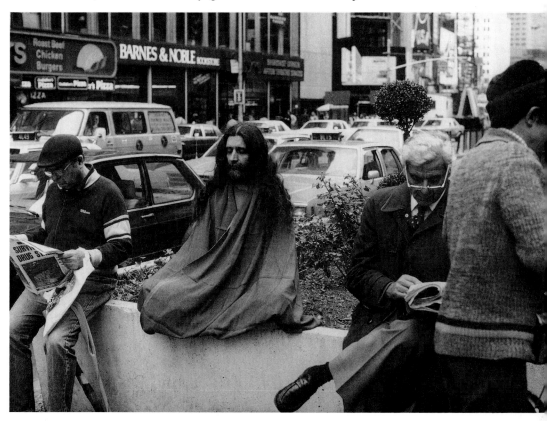

Prior to the North American Indian culture being crushed by European invaders, part of their cultural life involved being initiated into meditation and "mirroring the self" by different methods. The young Indian was then given a new name, which symbolically expressed both for himself and others the particular path that he had to follow to become more himself.

Traveling in Mexico and Columbia I have seen many sculptures that reveal evidence of meditation and yogic postures. On the Oseberg Viking ship in Norway you will find a bucket with the Lotus pose engraved in the handle; it is said to be of Irish or Celtic origin.

The debate over the power of words and thought - suggestion and *mantra* - is also not an exclusively Eastern phenomenon. In Scandinavia, too, sources indicate profound knowledge of these means and the effects they have. In the Finnish folk poems *Kalevala* are power words, primordial words, birth words; in Nordic folksongs we find the art of runes, sounds that have been known and used in the same way as the Indian mantras (see quotation on page 109).

In the Icelandic Edda manuscript it says, for example, that Odin was known as *Ome* among the gods. The word *OM* means sound in ancient Norse (*omr*) and in Sanskrit. Even today, in a Norwegian dialect, you find the word *om,* meaning "concentrated sound". In the Indian tradition *OM* is the symbol of the innermost, most fundamental sound or vibration. *OM* is often written *AUM* to be closer to how it is pronounced. The meaning of this word must have been universal as it reappears in the Judaic *AMEN*, in the Egyptian *AMON* (in the names of the pharaohs, for example, Tutankamon), in the Islamic *AMIN*. It is also said (for example, on the record "Les flûtes Indiennes") that flutes exist in both Egypt and South America that give the same sound and vibration as *OM*.

Knowledge that has been preserved about the psychic centres or *chakras* (which we will discuss in this book) is still a living tradition of the Hopi Indians. When the Dutch, according to the musician Dollar Brand, first landed on South African soil, they found people who meditated, though obviously the Europeans were completely unappreciative of this.

When it reached a certain stage of development, the church in Europe in an "all-knowing" manner began to suppress different ways of thinking, even within itself - and still does today - so that all such knowledge could only be handed down in secret societies. There has also been, however, a Christian form of meditation within certain monastic orders of the Catholic Church and especially the Greek Orthodox Church.

From all this we can conclude that we are dealing with a common human inheritance.

Yoga, Tantra and meditation is the science of man's body, mind and psyche. This knowledge contains concrete instructions on how to let go of physical and mental inhibitions. Evolution shows us that people today are intellectually and psychically prepared to accept much that even the last generation was hesitant about, and the reasons for applying this knowledge are obvious:

The development of the culture and of individual understanding

The information that science places at our disposal today, the attitude that psychology now takes about human potential and developments in art and thinking, all give new values and a new insight. And man is asking himself: how do I get in touch with my own potential and also become more open in my relationship with others?

Technical evolution

We may experience conflicts between the longing for inner freedom and strength and the ability to live with and participate in human society. Our desire is to be able to face any situation and still preserve inner peace, regardless of what happens around us. This depends often on how we perceive our world, and how we judge it.

Can we live in these times with all the problems and opportunities that surround us - and grow richer experiencing the multiplicity of life?

Psychic evolution

When you become conscious of yourself, when you open yourself and experience everything with increased sensitivity - then you must be able to receive the impressions from your environment and **experience** your own thoughts and feelings - even though these may come with ever-increasing strength.

The expansion of consciousness

Many who come to have an expansion of consciousness - either spontaneously or caused by sorrow and shock or through the use of certain drugs - are often not prepared to cope with such states. The effects can be multiple and different for each individual.

However, today consciousness is being expanded naturally in many different ways: people are learning to develop body awareness (heightened awareness of their own body and its movements), and are achieving a greater ability to tolerate thoughts and experience both their own and other people's feelings.

Psychic strength

Strength and psychic balance are attained through yoga and meditation. Research into breathing exercises, physical postures and various meditation techniques in laboratories around the world confirms the scientific validity of the yogi's experience.

Inspiration and meeting with life

Tensions can be relieved, depressions and lethargy disappear; but yoga and meditation are not only preventive and healing. New ideas come easier and we discover that our daily life has clarity and richness of content. Tantra makes it possible for you to live every moment **consciously** and to have a powerful, participating relationship with life.

Chapter 3

How to Begin...

When the need and interest arise, the question is: How do I get started?

This book is written both for those who want to begin on their own and for those who are already under way but want support and further instruction.

If you do not have any prior experience of yoga and meditation, do a few things regularly and patiently, rather than throwing yourself into an extensive training programme and expecting great accomplishments in an unreasonably short time.

Follow the instructions in this book carefully (nothing is included accidentally). If you are not sure about something, go back to it and work through it again. Do it as if for the first time, as if you don't know anything about the way it should be done.

The contents of the book are self-explanatory and are described in the next chapter as a suggested course of development.

You'll become acquainted with different exercises and programmes. For a harmonious result take one thing at a time, begin with the first exercises and go through them thoroughly. Do them regularly for a period of time, until you feel that you have mastered them and can do them without strain or restlessness.

Then follow the instructions, and go on to the next exercises. No exercise will be difficult if it is taken up when you have mastered the previous ones. This is also true of the meditation. Use the different methods. They don't cancel each other out but provide many paths towards the same goal - towards yourself, your own peace and strength.

In chapter 13 we take up the subject again regarding daily life. But first let us gain experience and gradually find the right amount - neither so much that the effort is troublesome nor so little that nothing comes of it. And remember: **You are doing this only because you want to, for your own needs**.

So why have a bad conscience if you don't achieve what you originally planned? Bide your time and start again when you feel like strengthening and exploring yourself.

Conditions

Are there any special conditions connected with meditating and using yoga?

Yes, ordinary common sense and a few rules such as not eating for three to four hours before doing yoga poses and breathing exercises and not doing them immediately after lying in the hot sun.

And if you want to take a bath, do it **before** and not after the exercises and meditation.

There are certain rules and certain restrictions for doing individual exercises, but these will be mentioned where appropriate.

Food

People often ask me if they have to eat special food to be able to practise yoga.

No! I feel good not eating meat and animal products, but that is my own personal taste and perception; it is not a condition. Keeping to a certain diet is a separate thing. You can get something out of yoga and you certainly can meditate no matter what you eat.

A good rule concerning diet is: don't eat too much, don't eat too little; and if now and then you don't feel like eating, skip a meal. It is said that the stomach should be one-quarter full in the morning, three-quarters full at noon and half full in the evening. And if you feel that a certain food makes you sluggish or nervous, avoid it.

The most important requirements are patience and a desire to go on; later, the effect of the exercises will inspire you and keep you going.

Yoga and meditation strengthen body and mind. Diet or fasting are only additions.

Yoga has a strong effect by itself.

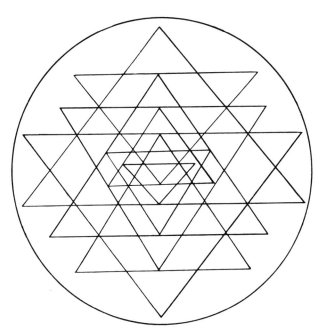

7

Chapter 4

8 Steps in Yoga and Meditation

...and a way to use this book

The fact that you have this book presumably means that you want to approach the subject in a practical way. You have decided to apply the system of yoga and meditation in your daily life.

So let's start. In the book you will find different facets of yoga described with guidance about how to use its methods.

In this chapter we will look at yoga and meditation as a process that will gradually prepare the body and mind for even deeper and finer methods and states. In this way, yoga grows and unfolds itself. Start with something that you feel is easy to do. But don't get stuck there. When you have used some of the physical exercises for some time and benefitted from them, then go on to others.

However, don't rush through the book. Development takes its own course. Even though you go forward and explore new aspects of yoga, it is important to deepen your knowledge of what you already know and use. When you start using yoga you may feel an effect right away, but give yourself time to let the effect become permanent and deeper.

You don't have to proceed through the book page by page, doing only one thing at a time. You can also use it as a handbook: survey the subject, then pick out a few things here and there, for example a programme of physical exercises, a breathing exercise, to be followed by a relaxation technique and perhaps a concentration exercise to use at another time of day.

We will discuss how you can proceed and prepare a regular daily training. In the chapter "Yoga for Daily Life" at the end of the book, we see that it becomes natural to use the exercises and to have more vitality. We benefit from the yoga and it fits into our day just like brushing our teeth, which is

incidentally a yogic exercise.

But first an overview, a progression through yoga and meditation - and through this book.

The eight steps are not theoretical in nature but a practical guide, not absolute laws or rules but simply a working draft, a suggestion about how development can be experienced.

Step 1/To discover the natural and free

Yoga is a powerful tool. It strengthens and sensitizes. If you put it to use, it will make you receptive and more creative.

The poses work by themselves through the body, and apart from peace the meditation gives insight and perspective. This step, like step 2, works best when it is used during the *Inner Silence* meditation, which is described in chapter 9.

Are you always ahead of life with expectations and demands? Do you feel frustrated - also with your own development and liberation? Or do you have time to stop and see what life really has to offer? Harmony is achieved when you see through your ideas and dreams, when you see through the "good" and "bad" and experience life as it is in itself - acting freely.

Why feel guilty?

Do you ever experience how your mood is affected by what you do and think?

Here is a practice for you:

Become aware of what influences you, the suggestions and invitations from your surroundings and from your world of thoughts.

What suggestions do I give myself, what offers do I take up, what decisions do I make? Do they point in the direction of greater openness and tolerance? Are my reactions based on anxiety, bad conscience and fear of criticism? Are my opinions and concepts acquired? Do I have principles that stop me from experiencing

and acting without having to wonder whether I am permitted - by others, by the group, the time, the fashion, the party, or my ideals?

Or do I get through to my inspiration, my real wishes and goals?

What inspires me to set about this task?

What gives my body and mind the best stimulation in the long run? What strengthens my desire and ability to meet with life?

Do you know how yoga and meditation exercises affect your frankness, your concentration and your scope?

What is it in particular that sometimes puts me in a very good mood?

Step 2 / To become conscious of what inhibits you

You may now expect that through yoga you will be in charge of your life, that you will have the capacity to control it and anticipate future events and avoid any surprises. And yet here I will suggest something else: Come to terms with the blocks that hinder you from living freely and harmoniously. Let go of your reservations when life turns out to be different from what you expected and join in.

Everything comes as suggestions: suggestions and proposals from the environment, from the body, from thoughts - see all that life offers you, all the suggestions that your impulses and your habits present you. Do not seek, but see them when they appear. Which do you *want* to follow?

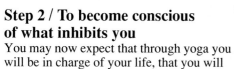

Which do you *actually* follow?

Can you experience yourself like a witness while you are angry, sleepy or sad - do you dare live it out, to be it? Can you act without making excuses? Or do you hide behind ideals and extreme demands on yourself and on the rest of us.

What about strong emotions - can one let oneself feel them, in the middle of daily life, can one let others see them? I am not talking about exhibiting oneself, or forcing oneself upon others.

Are there conflicts in your mind, reasons why you don't get done what you want to do, that so much pulls you, that time flies and nothing really happens?

First of all, **what you do anyway**, do it fully. Whatever you are doing, you can do it...

Sometimes I make plans that I never carry out. Can you distinguish between what you think, plan or dream and what you really do in your life? Do you normally do what you have decided, even the little, "unimportant" things? This is not the same as being stubborn and always insisting on doing things your way.

Do you, for instance, tire when someone hinders you from carrying out a plan, or when you don't get the job or task that you want, when you meet opposition or competition? Do you feel embittered?

Notice when something makes you dispirited or inhibits your actions. Yet do not cling to the experience or keep it at arm's length, but let it touch you; you are in the middle of it as long as it lasts, but no longer. Then go on.

Perhaps I am "forced" to be different people: one within the family, one in society, one at work, one when I'm alone with myself...

Can the different sides be collected in **one** person, is there a hidden split somewhere, is it possible to mend and unite the forces which pull in separate directions? Can one be whole, and live with all the opposites one contains?

Yes, one can - don't you want to face these opposites and be able to accept them? "I am this and I am also that".

And discomfort...

Do you feel discomfort?

Can you stay inside a feeling of discomfort, and experience it?

Do you often find yourself in a situation where you push aside discomfort and put the blame on someone or something else?

And in other similar situations, have you found that you repeat this?

To transform inhibitions

The method of opposite reaction is used especially in the beginning of the meditation, to prepare for the deeper states.

After all, I am not my thoughts. All that the mind reveals, it has a need to show. Dispirited thoughts must come up and out, be experienced. Only then the mind lets go of them and gives room to more positive thoughts.

Positive thoughts or suggestions that you put to yourself; the more deep-reaching and forward directed suggestions about what you really want - these appear when the mind has had the opportunity to finish thinking all the rest. When you relax while facing the thoughts, harmony and perspective appear of their own accord.

If your mind shows you negative suggestions and thoughts such as: "I'm miserable, it'll never work out"; "I'm ill"; "I don't want that"; "I'm nothing special"; etc., then be fully aware of them. Just let the thoughts come, as they are doing anyway - and look on while you're in that mood. But as soon as it is over and gone, be open to a positive suggestion, a good idea.

Follow the negative thought to the bottom, until it can go no further, until it looks quite hopeless - let the thought or emotion rage itself out - and then experience how the weak thought vanishes and a strong positive thought appears by itself. However, it's no good stopping halfway. Surrender to it, let it happen while you watch - all the way to the bottom. This is

a process that works over and over again. You do not seek or create any experiences, you just become conscious of the feelings and thoughts passing through your mind anyway.

Weakness is something one has grown used to over a long period of time. One breaks the habit by persistently using the same method for the same problem.

Let the negative suggestion be heard. After you have watched it take hold of you to such an extent that it exhausts itself, then a good idea and courage to face life itself will come. The negative and critical attitude is succeeded by a positive action.

Sitting with your hands in your lap does not remove depression or give concentration.

Yoga and meditation you do for your own sake and thus for everyone else, too. You need

both a certain atmosphere and the possibility to evolve. You surely prefer to do what you want in a relaxed and natural way. Therefore continue living the way that is natural for you - and let's take a look at step 3.

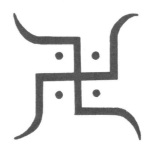

Step 3 / Physical well being

Health is something precious in itself. To achieve and maintain optimal health is the purpose of the yoga poses, but the poses also serve as an essential preparation for meditation.

Step 3 involves the physical exercises (*asana*) and their use. You get to know your own body, you move it, make it flexible and sensitive. With the yoga exercises, you work on the major areas of your body: the blood circulation, the muscles and organs, the glands and the digestive and nervous systems. So the poses are used to remove sluggishness of the bodily functions, psychosomatic problems and physical discomfort. Seen in the larger context of yoga, the *asana* relieve disturbances in the body which may cause trouble in the later steps. Chapter 6 and *Hatha Yoga* in chapter 5 discuss these exercises.

Here are two ways to work with the body. You should get to know both before you go on to the following steps of this chapter:

1. Start with exercises that are easy and make you supple. Discover the feeling of your body while you move it in an exercise and experience the form of your body when you hold it still. Then do the same with the more deep-working exercises - and feel the well being, sensitivity and strength that you attain in your sense organs, nervous system and breathing.

2. Now, sit totally still for longer periods of time and experience motionlessness in your body - in a chair, in a yoga pose, in one of the meditation poses.

Step 4 / The control of energy

When you feel confident about one programme and are gradually mastering its physical exercises, expand them with breathing exercises:

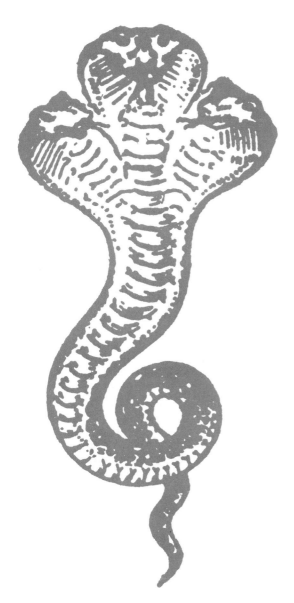

a. A few appropriate breathing exercises are mentioned right after the easier physical exercises. In these, you become aware of your breathing and you begin to learn to let your body breathe freely, without interfering.

b. Then you proceed to master your breathing and learn to release the blocks connected with it. This is done by working **regularly** on rhythmic breathing and the first stage of the real breathing exercises (*pranayama*).

c. When you have reached the more advanced physical poses, and only then, start using the corresponding breathing exercises with unfailing regularity, observing the instructions.

The breathing exercises provide you with the experience of the energy of the body and of the nervous system. You begin to control this energy and thus regulate tensions in your muscles, organs and nerves. It becomes easier to prevent diseases and depressions which are often caused by misplaced energy, physical, emotional and psychic - too much or too little tension in a part of your body. In India this energy is called *prana*. Around the world it has many names; the Austrian psychoanalyst Wilhelm Reich called it "orgone energy".

Your knowledge of how to control the psychic energy will grow gradually. It is called *Prana Vidya* (*vidya* = knowledge) and is also the name of an advanced Tantric healing method.

Most important about the breathing exercises is the liberating effect they have on the mind through the nervous system and the brain. The knowledge of the relationship between thought, tension and breathing is fundamental. Therapists and researchers who work with the body know that mental problems and memories are not stored in the brain alone, but in the whole body as muscle tension, inertia and insensitivity. By dissolving these inhibitions with yoga, the energy is again awakened, depressions are removed and emotions and memories, often reaching back to early childhood, are re-experienced.

Thomas Schmidt, a German doctor, has conducted research into the different relationships

between thinking and emotional activity of the mind and the way the body reacts to this activity (psychosomatic medicine). He has confirmed to me that every change in the way we breathe, its rhythm and speed, has a direct influence on the nervous system. Before learning of the breathing exercises in yoga, Dr. Schmidt concluded that, if one could influence the breathing consciously, one could create a very efficient therapeutic system. Today he knows that such a system already exists, and that it has been tested for thousands of years in yoga. It has evolved into a set of different breathing exercises, each one with specific effects.

The activity of the nervous system mainly consists of electrical and chemical impulses that should pass "fresh" sense impulses to the mind. As time goes on, however, cycles of inhibiting impulses are formed, which have a direct influence on the nervous system and the breath. These habits in the nervous system react completely automatically to certain experiences, emotions, or memories that you do not wish to recall. Thus high blood pressure, mental resistance or even depression is provoked and maintained. By regulating the breath or by systematically interfering with the breathing rhythm using different breathing exercises, these habitual cycles can be broken, the energy flows freely again and the brain is brought into a harmonic state.

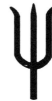

Step 5 / What about disturbances?

When you are under way with yoga and feel better, then you can meet life with greater openness and appreciate this step.

If you really want to meditate, learn a method which deals with the influences or disturbances affecting your senses and mind.

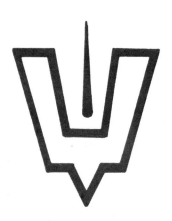

How do you experience disturbances: noises, smells, discomfort, pain? And your relationship to others - are people well- or ill-disposed towards you? Dare you be sensitive and accepting and open?

Have you tried just for a moment to experience in total all that happens around you? For a while drop all critical attitudes, don't reject anything - accept it all fully and partake in all that you see, hear and feel. And allow your mind to think all that you usually avoid. Don't fight it.

If you force the mind away from thoughts and disturbances, it will always return to them. *Pratyahara* counts on the mind's reaction. You satisfy the mind's need and concentration becomes possible. This method from the Tantric tradition is described in chapter 9.

A practical example of Pratyahara is also given along with the Back Stretch and Abdominal Stretch poses on pages 74 and 76. Pratyahara forms the transition from yoga to meditation, leading you to deep relaxation and true concentration.

All the steps so far are called **indirect**: by removing difficulties, diseases and disturbances, they are intended to prepare the body and mind for concentration. The last three steps are called **direct**: you turn your attention to the essential - how to concentrate, meditate, become one with yourself and what you do.

Step 6 / Concentration

When you are no longer buffeted about by thoughts and emotions, when the periods of concentration become more frequent, more permanent and stable, then you will proceed naturally to this step, which I call "inspired interest": to be absorbed, or to act, without losing inspiration, and without becoming either restless or dispirited...

You learn to keep your attention on what you want. This reflects back: when you remove your interest and energy from tensions in body and mind, you cannot hold the tensions. This has a healing effect (chapter 10).

Step 7 / Meditation

Meditation is being able to rest in a deeply relaxed state and from that gather energy and perspective.

It is to be conscious with a clear awareness, inner as well as outer. Clarity means the capacity openly to meet any experience and remain yourself (chapter 11).

Step 8 / To live fully

To achieve a genuine rest in yourself: what does that really imply? Is it something mystical and unworldly or is it a real, present possibility? To be yourself under all conditions in such a harmonious state that you also feel a part of, and in harmony with, the universe and with life, or - as many have expressed and experienced it - with the divine within yourself and in everything, so that nothing is alien to you?

You express and accept your thoughts, feelings and actions. When something has already happened, what help is it to regret or suffer? When holiness, charity or even righteousness become ideals, then they lose their true quality. You don't have to wear a mask or adhere to form. You live now, straightforwardly and without posing for others (methods, chapter 12).

Conclusion

The understanding of what lies behind these eight steps is achieved through practice. It is not only a question of proceeding from one step to the next - rather, think of all the steps (even step 8) as separate entities that gradually can be used side by side. For the yogi, development takes place by ceaselessly moving back and forth within these steps - using what is described in the following chapters.

Return to this chapter when you have really started to use the different practices. You will then see these 8 steps in the light of the experiences you have gained.

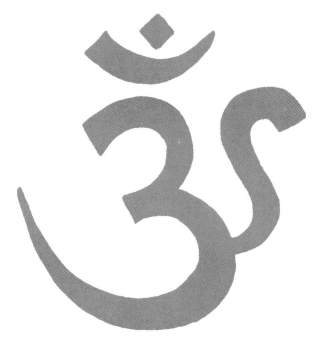

Chapter 5

The Different Spheres of the Yogic Tradition

What have we inherited from the past and how can we use it?

Can I see through the prejudices and limitations of the past and develop a personal and living relationship to these yoga techniques and psychological methods? After all, I am not seeking a ready-made world view and I am not interested in learning a lot of technical terms or letting myself be converted.

If we want an understanding of how yoga and meditation can enrich our lives, then we can hardly avoid the four or five great classical branches of yoga or the essentials of the science at the root of these, namely Tantra. In this chapter we will also touch upon other concepts from India: the ashram, the swami tradition, the chakras and so forth.

This will not be a complete dissertation on what has been said and written about these subjects but rather a description of what is innermost and characteristic, inspiring and useful about them.

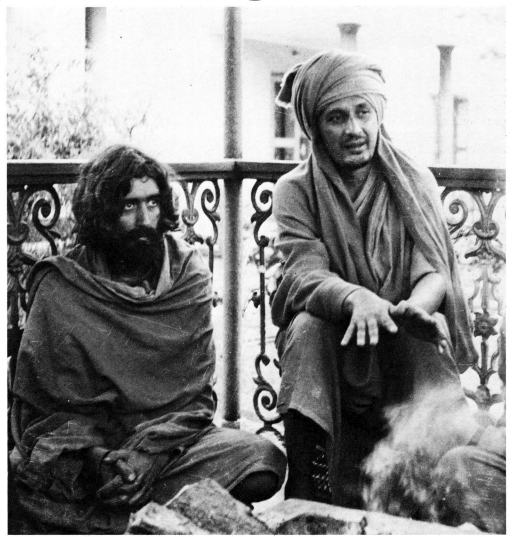

The spiritual attitude is over and over again to restore the connection with the great harmony.
(Swami Satyananda)

Yoga is traditionally divided into a number of branches. *Hatha Yoga* is concerned with the balance and mutual influence of the physical and the psychic/mental. *Karma Yoga* uses activity to overcome inhibitions and apathy: you set yourself a definite goal, undertake a task, and work steadily to achieve that task. Still it is not the fruit or result which is important, nor the worry about it, but consciousness in the act - experience and awareness. *Raja Yoga* is the knowledge of the mind and of the laws that limit and liberate it. In Tantra, Raja Yoga acquires practical expression in the various methods and meditations. *Jnana Yoga* is about how to realize your own essence and being. To develop discrimination - to confront the states and powers in you, and behind the deep rooted ideas about your limitations, to become one with your true identity. The result is an integrated personality. *Bhakti Yoga* is possibly the most difficult; it is about devotion.

From one stand-point, Hatha Yoga is part of Raja Yoga.

These branches are four sides of the same whole. We might also call them: wisdom, insight, enlightenment and innocence.

Hatha Yoga

Hatha Yoga springs from the teaching about the two sides of our being: the ability to act and the ability to reflect.

Ha is symbolized by the sun, the warm, creative and physical side of our being, *Tha* by the moon, the cool, receptive and psychic side.

This old principle of the sun and the moon, can be compared with two functions of the nervous system, the sympathetic and the parasympathetic.

When the relationship between **psyche** and **soma**, between thoughts/emotions and body/tension/energy is not in balance, when both these nervous functions, which have to respectively inhibit/calm or quicken/awaken the body, are working against each other, then we are dealing with stress and psychosomatic disorders. Nervous diseases, ulcers, catarrh, diabetes, certain types of constipation and other physical illnesses, often have an emotional and mental origin or are brought about by a failing ability to handle conditions of the environment (stress).

The purifying processes of Hatha Yoga create a foundation that maintains a harmonious balance in the body. Your mind and your ability to concentrate and unfold in life is influenced by impurities and tensions. When they are removed you experience the deeper causes. Therefore, Hatha Yoga is the beginning of physical yoga and combines with the physical poses (*asana*) and breathing exercises (*pranayama*) to cure and prevent psychosomatic diseases. Yoga keeps the body alive and vital despite age, and keeps your metabolism in order and improves your concentration. Your circulation is stimulated by blood-pumping exercises and through gravity when the body is in an upside-down pose. The nervous system is strengthened especially by breathing exercises. The functions of the glands are regulated through cleansing processes and poses which, in themselves, also affect the general condition of the body.

First the organs of the body have to be cleansed, thereby discarding their sluggishness. Sediments in the alimentary canal and in the glandular ducts must be removed. Hatha Yoga itself consists of only six cleansing processes. In Sanskrit these six processes are called *shat karma* or *kriya* (not to be confused with *Kriya Yoga*):
1. Neti, a process of purifying and strengthening the entire nasal passage and making it more sensitive. There are different variations (page 56).
2. Dhauti, a series of different techniques to cleanse the alimentary canal from mouth to anus. These also include techniques to cleanse the eyes, ears, teeth, tongue and scalp.
3. Nauli, a very powerful method of massaging and strengthening the lower abdomen and intestines (page 57).
4. Basti, techniques for washing and strengthening the colon.
5. Kapalabhati, techniques for purifying the front part of the brain (page 56).
6. Tratak, a process whereby you look intensely at an object for increasing lengths of time to develop your concentration and the dormant psychic powers that we all possess. It is a very effective eye exercise which relaxes the eyes and the brain (page 103).

Swara Yoga

In Swara Yoga we are taught to experience and control the relationship between sun and moon. Swara Yoga is an independent part of yoga, related to Hatha Yoga and *Kundalini Yoga*.

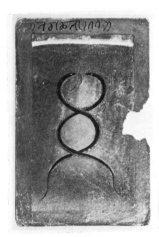

In the spinal cord, according to the timeless Tantric and yogic sciences, there exist three main currents. The central current, going through the middle of the spinal cord, is called *Sushumna,* "the direct way home". It opens during meditation and brings power to the brain which it activates. At that time both nostrils will be fully open. This power, known as Kundalini, is not awakened, neither partially nor fully, if there is no balance between the two other currents in the spine: the *Ida* (moon) and *Pingala* (sun).

Normally your two nostrils are open at different times and, if not prevented for example by disease or by mental troubles, they alternate very regularly. For about one hour and twenty minutes, one nostril opens completely and the other closes, and then after a further hour and twenty minutes, the reverse happens. Hold the upper side of one hand under one nostril and then under the other and feel by the flow of air which of your nostrils is more open right now.

Psychophysiologists have become aware of this phenomenon and are now investigating the relationship between the different characteristics of the two sides of the brain and the air flow in the nostrils. The descriptions given today of the functions of the two brain halves and the knowledge preserved in the yoga tradition concerning *Ida* and *Pingala* agree closely. In yoga not only the brain but the whole central nervous system and thus the whole body is taken into account.

The Swara yogi is aware of which of the nostrils is opened and when. For example, intellectual and social work is benefited if the left one is open. On the other hand if a meal is to be properly digested and if the body is to perform some physical or creative work, then the more energetic right nostril should be open.

This is a very brief description, but more details are preserved in yogic tradition. By regulating the nostrils, you can avoid becoming too introspective and gloomy or on the other hand too insensitive or physically violent.

It is thought possible to predict the significance and outcome of different events by checking the nostrils' breathing in relation to what is happening.

Swara Yoga reveals the presence of *Ida* and *Pingala* and their functions. The two currents flow from *Muladhara Chakra* (the lowest

placed major chakra in the body), through the spinal cord to *Ajna Chakra* (the chakra found behind the eyebrow centre in the middle of the head), crossing each other at every chakra.

Certain yogis keep the left nostril (moon) open during the day, and at night they sleep on their left side, so that the right (sun) nostril is uppermost and therefore open.

Kundalini Yoga

How can this energy lying dormant within us be awakened? How can we benefit fully from it?

When harmony exists between intellect and intuition, between mind and body, between body and emotions, when *Ida* and *Pingala* are in balance and the central current in the spine, the *Sushumna*, is opened, when the force rises and awakens the chakras, then we talk about Kundalini Yoga. Then the brain becomes fully awake, our potential flourishes and we become aware of our states - we experience deep insight and harmony.

Physiology has taught us that we only use between 10 and 20 percent of the brain's capacity. The rest belongs to the subconscious or the unconscious, and abilities present in those areas lie dormant, idle, unused.

Why are we so limited, why isn't full vitality at our disposal from the very start? We might just as well ask why a flower must first be a bud or a butterfly a pupa. Life is obviously experienced as a growing process. Little by little we gain abilities and energy. One day this development will compel you to awaken the power consciously and acquire the freedom it gives you - that is the purpose of the methods in Kundalini Yoga.

There are different methods at our disposal. But first we must be aware of how the psychic energy acts here and now. We begin by penetrating our habitual tensions and thoughts, becoming sensitive and aware, deepening our state. We have seen how

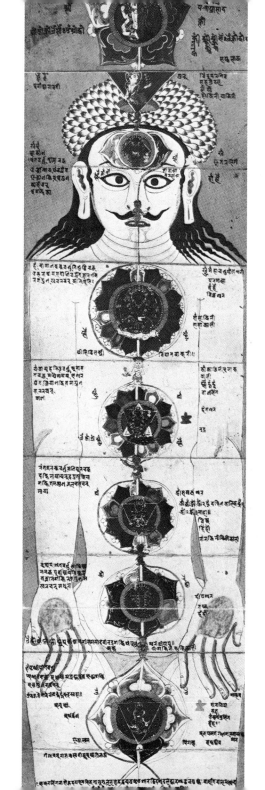

physical yoga helps us. Kundalini Yoga also uses the yoga exercises. The Plough, the Shoulderstand, the Fish, the Spinal Twist, to name a few, through their physical influence awaken the energy fields of the chakras; and the experience of the energy is made possible through the use of the breathing exercises; altogether they give you a fundamental knowledge of the chakras.

Obviously Hatha Yoga and the physical poses can be used for health and beauty aids, but beauty also comes from within and you get something extra into the bargain, an insight into the psyche - psychic strength.

Behind everything we experience there is psychic energy. How you conceive of it is up to you, it depends on your expectations, wishes, problems - on your entire character.

When you experience the intensity of this energy, it may lead you to get involved and create associations with personal emotions or thoughts. If you feel sadness or fear, if you experience enthusiasm, you may think it has an outer cause and depends on the actual situation you find yourself in at the time.

The realization that states, emotions and thoughts need not have an "external" cause, that they may express a fundamental inherent power - energy from different layers of the psyche that you unconsciously identify with - is the beginning of Kundalini Yoga. Thoughts and emotions are seen through and that which lies behind is contacted and experienced at the chakras (see chapter 8).

Raja Yoga

Raja Yoga is the royal road or the knowledge of the mind.

"Yoga dissolves the barriers of the mind", it is said at the beginning of the Yoga Sutras, a manuscript written by Rishi Patanjali 2300 years ago.

When you work with the mind and realize its laws, when you meditate and use the

methods that overcome the limitations of the mind, when you master the inclinations of the mind with a firm and steady concentration, then you walk the royal path; you are using Raja Yoga, the ancient psychology.

Raja Yoga is a methodical science, a science that can be acquired. It is not possible to know all at once, not even about your own mind - to view its depths and know its laws. This knowledge therefore is preserved and passed on from generation to generation.

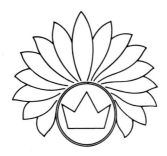

You can master a mad elephant;
You can close the mouth of a bear or tiger;
By alchemy you can earn your bread;
You can wander incognito throughout the
*   universe;*
Make the gods your slaves and preserve
*   eternal youth;*
You can walk on water and live in fire;
But - to control your mind is better and more
difficult.   (Thayumanavar)

Raja Yoga is about concentration, although it must be effortless so that it does not lock you up but opens you.

In Raja Yoga the concentrated states are defined, the different possibilities and abilities are explained, along with the many obstacles to be avoided. It contains a charting of human nature and psyche, defining its three temperaments: 1. the light and clear, full of insight; 2. the active and passionate; and 3. the dull and self-forgetful.

But Tantra says, "Rise by that which makes you fall." If you can cause inertia in yourself,

you can also master it and that is better than suppressing it. Then you can go further.

In Tantra, Raja Yoga is primarily of a practical nature: it offers concrete methods to fool the mind's reactions, cleverly worked out techniques capable of rousing and holding attention.

In practice Tantra does not distinguish between the different branches of yoga; they form a whole. And you will find Raja Yoga throughout this book - the entire sequence is based on it.

Bhakti Yoga

Bhakti is the art of devotion -
to live life always unfolding,
fulfilling your destiny,
as an act of devotion.

To be able to live and act in life, to be
able to give yourself to it and do what
you do without second thoughts or doubts
is Bhakti.
Don't think twice
it is all right
all acts are as they are
all thoughts are allowed
conforming to your own deepest way
of perceiving things
conforming to the whole of which you
yourself are a part.

To feel secure with what is now,
existing, living, being at home here,
is Bhakti.

To write about Bhakti is something special,
to write about
being able to throw yourself into life
firmly anchored in devotion,
so that every action is done without a doubt
so that everything you do
you do
because it is your way

of expressing by devotion
the innermost
or highest
will.

To sing is Bhakti, God's name, or what
you experience as
exalted, to read poetry about it,
is Bhakti,
but Bhakti is most of all
to live a normal life
with normal work, and to experience **that**
like a poem -
life and work is the homage to
God, to life, to the whole
to the innermost and truest in you and me.
And everything I do, that I can do
that I can do...
That I do -
That I do.

Karma Yoga

For the Karma yogi it is more thrilling to
solve a problem, accomplish a task, or even
rid himself or herself and others of physical or
psychic distress, than to be entertained - if
you throw yourself into a task then there is
not much time left over. What looks from the
outside like a struggling person involved only
with work, is in reality someone very inspired
and attentive, absolutely clear-headed about
what he/she is doing.

I like what I do...

I look on the whole of life as a creative
process. It takes place before my eyes, and I
am part of it - I am the witness and the
participant.

The more I give myself to my task, the less
I think about my own comfort or discomfort,
the more I feel part of something that is not just
about me, but about all of us - about everything.

To unfold myself, and to do it in a way that
will benefit not only me - that is the meaning
of life itself. In this way the Karma yogi
achieves freedom.

The Karma yogi's aid in this is awareness,
enhanced and trained by the inner intensity of
a daily meditation, *and* by being present with
open eyes in the midst of life's actions. Every
day I realize how to rely on myself and not be
carried away by how tasks "should" be done,
I solve them on the basis of what I really
believe, on the basis of the moment - the now.

Emotions, thoughts, wishful thinking, cravings,
anger - and the worries that follow - are seen
through, accepted and exhausted in the act.

In the now, in the unbroken sequence of
nows, I find life and opportunities to enjoy,
feel happiness, feel pain and anger -
everything that is me, everything that I do.
Going on...

Be attentive - experience
one: outer influences (people, sounds, music,
writings, images, talk, traffic, etc.)
two: spontaneous and habitual thoughts
three: yourself - with all this, in this and
without it.

Your life - what you are doing now,
your work when you're working
- is the object of your meditation.
Live it fully, the way **you** want to and
pay attention to **one, two, three.**

Karma Yoga is the ability to start all over again
- any time - and to continue the work. You
don't let yourself get knocked out or carried
away by how things are turning out.

And anyway there is nothing called yoga -
it's called life.

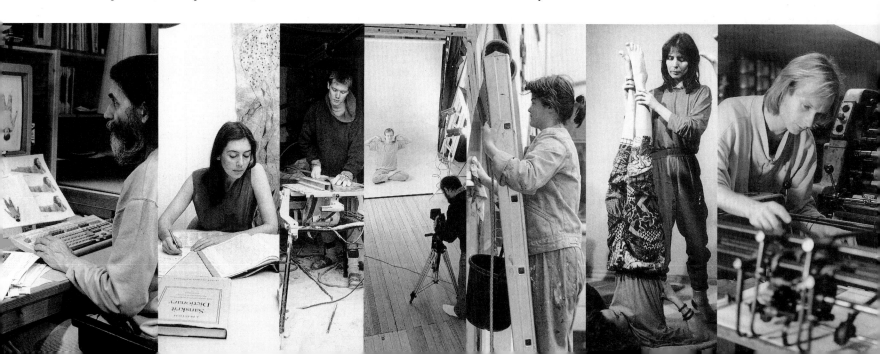

Karma

The word Karma is often misinterpreted to mean what is unavoidable in "life" or "fate". "An Indian farmer doesn't plough his land according to modern methods, since he considers that it is his Karma to be poor."

This has nothing to do with the objective concept of Karma in the Tantric or yogic science. Karma stands for everything that you were not conscious of, what you have partially experienced without fully comprehending, without really confronting or seeing it for what it is.

Things, people, you or me, whatever - be it inner or outer experiences - are seldom experienced for what they are but rather **what we consider** them to be.

When are we on an equal footing, understanding, accepting, generous? When do we consider ourselves better than others, wiser? When do we consider ourselves smaller, inferior, worshipping...?

What are the situations and people we experience really like? We think we know. Of course we know our friends and family, we might say, and then we expect them to behave accordingly. But do we really know?! Or we fantasize (in thoughts, dreams, etc.) how others are, the other group, people, society - even yoga. And how often do we dream about being somebody rather than finding out how we really are? Reality in itself is fine, but we expect something other than what is there. We get out of touch and suffer from a conflict, with consequences we may not even see.

Everything not understood, or rather not experienced for what it is, frustrates us consciously, or even worse unconsciously, since it does not live up to our expectations, to our wishes and ideals. On this basis our attitudes and habits are formed or reinforced, influencing the way we act, the situations we get into, what we radiate, how we affect our surroundings. And it is these attitudes, towards ourselves, our lives and towards others that determine whether we live a happy or an unhappy life. This, briefly, is what Karma stands for.

The "law" of Karma, our unconscious, seeks to bring us into situations where we can carry out the resolutions and wishes which were not fulfilled, where we can re-experience what we did not understand before, whatever caused us to react or idolise, what we did not see on an equal footing. That is the law of action and reaction.

Bad actions form bad Karma, good actions form good Karma - who can make a distinction? If I lie, it will certainly affect me more or less unconsciously. I lie to avoid something, something I don't want to face; perhaps I lie to myself and thus I can't see the consequences of the lie - a so-called vicious circle is formed... I get a "bad" conscience and that affects my self-image and my surroundings. A "good" action on the other hand gives me some satisfaction and thus peace of mind. But both "good" and "bad" actions create Karma!

The Karma of the yogi, on the other hand, is neither good nor bad. The yogi sees, experiences, and confronts everything with great awareness - sees it as it is, never judges. Nothing is either attractive or repulsive, it simply is. He creates no future Karma, either good or bad, he simply lives.

Karma Yoga can be seen from this interpretation of the word Karma.

Right or left, black or white. What *is* it that you must do? It is all about you, your Self - in our great totality. Shine!

Jnana Yoga

If you want a mirror,
look at this moment - respectfully.

When you have learned to experience, without trying to hold on to events, thoughts and emotions, but to let them come and go of their own accord...

When you have learned to perceive the automatic processes in your mind, habits in your life style, in the patterns of your thoughts and emotions, and accept what you experience without feeling guilty and without suppressing what you experience...

When you have taught yourself to be naked, not to clothe yourself in ideals or cravings for being holy, good and just...
then it will all become much easier, both for you and for us...
then you will discover real calm, full energy and richness in your actions, and you will experience oneness with yourself.

Jnana Yoga is pointing in that direction.

In Tantra there are two ways of reaching the witnessing awareness behind your acting and participating person, two seemingly contradictory attitudes:

I am not what I experience, I am the one experiencing it. I am not my body, thoughts, reputation, opinions, knowledge, emotions, name, senses, will - I am consciousness, at rest in itself. In the meditation *Inner Silence* we use this attitude. See chapters 9 and 12.

The other attitude is: **I am all this.** I am part of everything and everything is part of me. All that I experience, I am - now. And if someone says that I am such and such, I say: Yes, I am that too. I am all that, everything that happens within me and outside me.

This Tantric method does not run away from anything. If you feel ambition, you realize it, and exhaust it in your Karma Yoga, so that others may benefit from it too. Or you give it a symbolic name, which you become one with in your meditation. *Durga* is used in India, for example, as an expression for the force behind actions. If the most profound anxiety, the very darkest blackness threatens, then you go to meet it, and allow yourself to be invaded by it till you become one with it. Or else - like an Indian who identifies with the terrifying goddess *Kali* - you can hold it in a symbolic form, so that you avoid suppressing it or turning it into unconscious tension. Whatever you experience, accept it, become one with it; thus it is changed into inner security. You become the one you are, and nothing else but what you are. You become yourself.

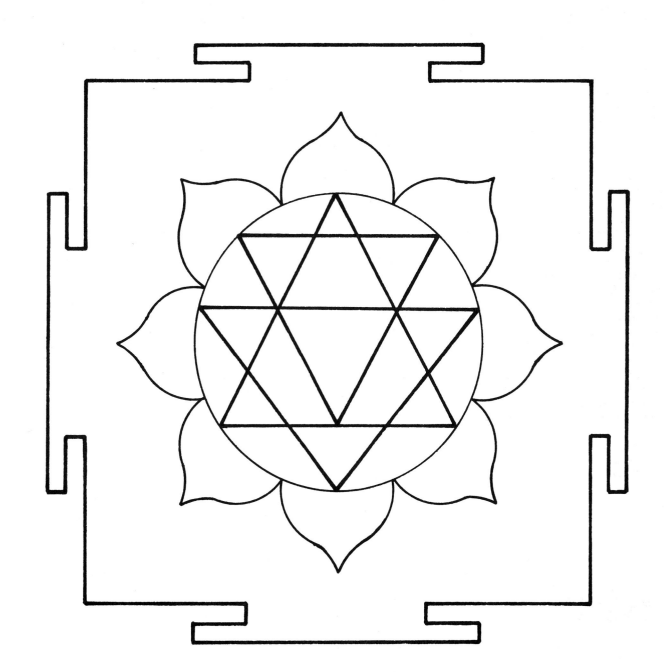

Different cultures may have different symbols, but the essence is the same: to find a symbol or a form that lets you experience reality and the power at work behind it - does it enchant you or are you there yourself?

"I am not the thoughts, the events. I am the experiencer"; or "I am all this": two formulas whose philosophical or other meaning is of no significance. It is not the interpretation which is important, but that they trigger a process in your mind which makes it possible for you to experience yourself as consciousness.

Tantra

Tantra is a conscious method of liberating man. The meaning of the word shows how: *tanoti* means to expand and *trayate* to liberate. By expanding your understanding of the depths of your mind, you become the master of it. By expanding your knowledge and insight you gain freedom, but only when the insight is based on your own experience.

Symbols

The concept of dualism is the starting point in Tantra, therefore also in yoga, as we saw in Hatha Yoga and Swara Yoga: a dualism in which the two sides are parts of a single whole.

Dualism is polarity or tension between matter/energy and consciousness, between positive and negative poles. A certain tension must be there for something to happen (electricity, human relationship, creation). Symbolically this is expressed as the relationship between and the union of *Shiva* and *Shakti* - the passive (experiencing) consciousness △, the masculine, and the creative (acting) force ▽, the feminine.

In reality you are both, because if there were no energy, there would be nothing to experience, and without consciousness there is no experiencer ✡.

Tantra therefore contains no idealism, but symbols to make tangible the fundamental states in the human being, e.g. fear, sorrow, enthusiasm of a superficial or deeper kind. Limitations and inhibitions of the human being are discovered, accepted/allowed and exhausted/relaxed.

Symbols are used by religious people as objects of veneration to strengthen their ideas of the universe. But symbols can also be abstract. To someone who has left organized religions and who may also be an atheist, symbols stand for archetypes in the mind's unconscious, fundamental thought forms whose energy can be released and put to use. At the same time, symbols express laws of the mind, like signposts and keys to open the doors of the mind.

Capacity, motive and decision

Tantra is considered the substructure of yoga. It is based on a **written** tradition, 64 Tantric *shastras*, and on an **oral** transmission, which is more important. Without the personal contact between teacher and student the books are worthless.

The real truth is hidden from one who is unable to show perseverance and trust, who cannot enter into the demanding collaboration and shared life that such a relationship involves. Not everyone has matured, there are those who must continue to live in the illusion that they know - their opinions all culled from fine books. Superficial knowledge and loads of facts hinder the ability to allow an unexpected experience and prevent one from acting in a way not previously planned.

The capacity to let go, therefore, is one of the most important requirements. A sufficient maturity must have been attained by the student in order for him or her to conceive of a greater context than his/her limited personal one, and truly to accept freedom in all areas of life. Whether you have a teacher or whether life is your teacher, you will never get anywhere unless you can see and listen and be receptive.

But when are you ready? Maybe when you are motivated. When you have seen that you can make something of your life, give it new horizons and break out of old ruts. In human growth itself there is an unconscious decision and purpose - *sankalpa*. Whatever you may think or want, it involves a direction.

The direction determines your growth. This direction can be influenced by a **conscious** resolution. It is such a resolution that activates you. The decision, the motivation and the desire determine the direction. The desire to move on and go further - the desire to grow and mature still more. In chapter 2 we talked about different reasons or motives for using Tantra; here we're talking about the basic decision - the driving force behind your work.

Sadhana

But how do you make a resolution so that it works, so that it is not destroyed by the re-actions of the mind, by old ideas of what you can or cannot do? Here we have a circle. We decide to get started and the work cleanses and relaxes the mind so that the resolution can work in depth - deeper than any doubt - and then it becomes easier to continue the work.

Make the resolution when you are most relaxed, when you lie in deep rest, in *Yoga Nidra* (chapter 9), and formulate it in such a way that you take it for granted.

We must, however, follow up the resolution and the desire with meditation and exercises. What shall we use to strengthen our concentration and where shall we go easy? Which tendencies of the mind shall we choose to exhaust?

Sadhana is the awareness of working with oneself, of being able to relax and concentrate at the same time, to strive without becoming rigid.

In the Tantric science and European Gnosticism, one talks about three temperaments or life attitudes that dominate a person (see also under Raja Yoga). Sometimes one, sometimes another, sometimes the third dominates. The three are called:

1. the dull and unconscious, the "bound" or "material";
2. the active, competent, the "heroic" or "physical";
3. the rich in insight and experience, the "godly" or "spiritual".

Organized religions and earlier generations, in their idealism and their attempts to purify, often made the mistake of imprisoning the human personality and its potential, thus preventing its different sides or temperaments from gaining expression: it was incarcerated in the dominating ideal.

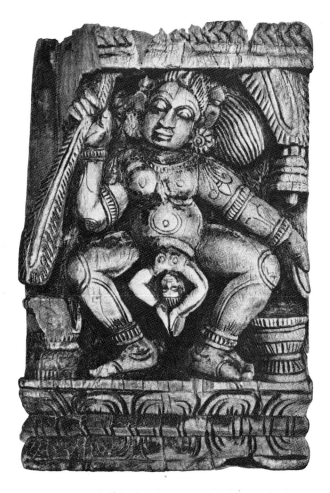

But the human being is not a schematic model, in a system that has been contrived: it is alive, subject to change and therefore it is dominated by different forces at different times. Whatever technique or way of life is suitable for the occasion, the teacher and one's own intuition can be of help. Every new situation is experienced for itself, not judged according to a preconceived scheme.

Ritual and meditation
The state that is elevated, deep and free... is the common goal of meditation and ritual. In Tantra both have a dynamic sequence as form.

The sequence and its components must hold the mind unceasingly; concentration must never fail, the mind should never become bored; interest must be held, the ability to go with the experience and remain open must be kept alive. And there must be a development, in which step-by-step you go deeper so at last you experience the fine states that we are tempted to call "dreamlike light", though they are fully conscious and full of power.

The ordinary waking state is preoccupied with our sense experiences. Inside we are preoccupied with thoughts and emotions and maybe inner psychic experiences. The meditative state, on the other hand, contains fewer impressions, is less preoccupied and more filled by consciousness in itself, by peace and perspective. The sequence leads us this way.

The Karma yogi's life is also a ritual, a way in which activity conquers all the little things that bury a person - self-pity, worry, complexes and neuroses. By turning the mind to the task and holding it steady in the here-and-now, these limitations are avoided.

The sequence is a process that inevitably holds the mind so that it does not yield to its own weakness. In a sense, this kind of ritual has a therapeutic function, but reaches further and higher than most therapies.

Different rituals master fundamental life situations: sex (chapter 7), death, loneliness and the responsibilities of family and society. These rituals are astoundingly effective.

Basic elements
Tantra, mantra, yantra, and nada - the method, the name, the form, the sound. *Tantra* is the method we will use. *Mantra* is the name, syllable or word used to get in contact with the mind. *Yantra* is the form we hold in our mind when we go deeper, a symbol that helps us to distinguish the mind from its contents. *Nada* is the sound that appears when the mind refrains from clinging to its tensions, when it lets thoughts flow freely and gives the body a chance to relax from within. The sound is experienced when the mind is naturally concentrated.

The name, the form and the sound are three sides of the same thing.

The name is your real name - what your mind answers to and feels secure with. By using this sound, you create a vibration that strengthens and relaxes the mind. The name is called mantra. It is derived via Sanskrit from the Indo-European words *man* (to think, from manas: mind) and *tra* (trayate, to liberate).

There are many different mantras with different effects. Just as colours more superficially affect the mind, so you can influence your mind by repeating or using a mantra when you meditate.

Often the sounds in a mantra are combined for an added symbolic meaning. They can provide a conscious level for you to become one with. They give a name to a form that you can relate to. But it is the sound in itself that has an effect by its vibrational frequency, its vibration and colour; the meaning is in addition to that, especially when several syllables are combined. The mantra that we use in chapter 11, *SO-HAM*, consists of two abstract seed syllables, each having an effect on the mind, one when you inhale, the other when you exhale. This enables you to contact and relax areas in your subconscious or unconscious, and gather your mind. The mantra has been given a meaning as well as this abstract effect; *So-Ham* "I am he" or *Sa-Ham* "I am she". I am my own essence, I am the all - consciousness, the universe,

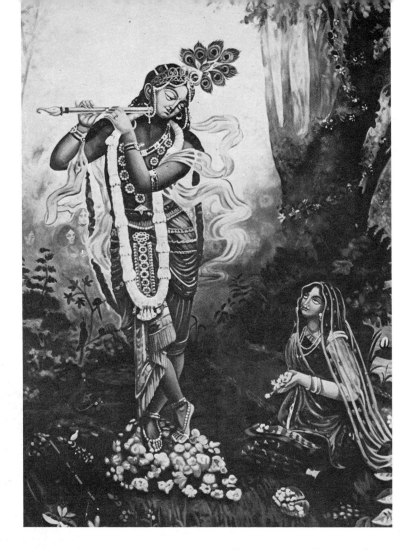

Yantra, or forms, are not only symbols of thought power, they also **produce** this power: a certain form causes an echo in the unconscious and corresponds to a certain effect.

Choose your symbol in deep meditation after you have learned the different methods in this book. Let the symbol appear by itself, don't think about wanting to understand it, just experience it - and once you have chosen, stick to that form. Shifting from one symbol to another only creates confusion in the mind. And don't talk about it at all if you want to keep its intensity.

The sound is that sound you can hear in yourself when the mind has reached a certain level of relaxation, a certain state. If you reach to the depths with the help of a mantra, you will be able to hear that vibration which the mantra symbolizes as a sound.

When your mind is steadily fixed on a yantra, the sound will arise from the area in the consciousness that you thus relax. If you do yogic poses and breathing exercises, the mind will become relaxed.

At a certain point you will be so finely attuned that you will hear the vibrational frequencies of the levels of consciousness to which you open yourself.

But the sound can also be contacted more directly, just as you can concentrate directly on an object. To do this methodically is known as *Nada Yoga*. It is not difficult; you just have to know the method. When you hear these sounds, let everything else flow past, let go, let the mind rest in the sound (nada). But the sound is not just **one** sound, it is different sounds that appear one or more at a time.

When you contact **one** stratum of consciousness, a corresponding sound, or type of sounds, will come; when you contact what is heard behind the first sound, you go deeper - through the various levels of consciousness, in toward your self.

In the following chapters we will go into the practical use of these fundamentals in the meditation techniques.

primal force. By meditating on this meaning, the mind can also let itself be brought to a greater experience of wholeness. But you are free to use this name with a meaning or only as an abstract vibration.

The form is your innermost form, symbol of your being - a thing, image, diagram, geometric figure that you have chosen to hold onto during your meditation. The mind is elusive and may contain anything. One thing may be hard to distinguish from another. By visualising the form, you are in a position to perceive the mind as an object, as something you can experience.

The form is called yantra. *Yan* means to retain (in a form), *tra* to liberate. You choose one object to keep your mind fixed on, and everything else that enters or surfaces in the mind need not trouble or trap you - you are one with the form and you let the rest go by. You don't have to strain or try to control any experience. The mind becomes one-pointed and restlessness no longer has a hold on you.

Meditative Song and Being Together

Kirtan

Song and dance are deeply rooted in all cultures. We find elevating songs and ecstatic dances all over the world. Certain of these songs and dances changes the state of awareness in a way similar to meditation. The best known of these are the American Indian sun dance, Sufi dancing in Arabic countries and the kirtan in India. And we find different kinds of music with healing effects from Africa to Greenland.

Everyone can participate in a kirtan. Unlike the bhajan, the kirtan is an unorthodox, popular, free form of expression. We take a mantra, for example *OM Anandam*, and a melody which we sing over and over. Thus the mantra gains power and the vibrations affect the mind, which vibrates with it.

One person who plays and sings the melody often leads the kirtan, or we let go of the fixed form and mantra and give in to a free music, where everybody plays, sings or dances.

If you continuously participate in this unfolding and stay with it all the time without reservation, you liberate yourself in the movements and the music.

When you succeed in this, you will experience a strong spontaneous relaxation in the meditation at the end of the music - and that will give you a starting point to understand some of the essence of meditation.

Satsang

Satsang means being together with one who rests in himself (*sat* means being) or communicating with those who are in the process of discovering this.

Satsang strengthens your motivation and makes it easier to keep alert.

In connection with a yoga and meditation training, it is common practice to attend satsang at which students gather around their teacher.

Some consider satsang to be the most important part of a sadhana. Different subjects are discussed, problems brought up, questions asked, perhaps about an aspirant's sadhana or about his or her way of living or about how meditation and yoga can be fitted into everyday life.

Satsang may be held every evening or only occasionally.

Often the teacher gives brief, perceptive answers. You may not understand the whole meaning at once, your mind has to work with it a while before you can take it all in. But the student always feels inspired in one way or another and the teacher equally becomes inspired by his student to continue with the work.

Satsang ends with a group meditation which is either instructed or silent.

Ashram

Ashram means workshop.

The workshop is the place where you find your form of work.

When you discover what that is all about, the ashram is your base for a longer time or just for a while.

A workshop is a complete unit always buzzing with the activity and group tasks that such mini-societies have: planning, food preparation, classes, studies, meditation, instruction of yoga teachers, giving various courses.

In my experience, excessively strict rules are not emphasized, but working norms are set and adhered to, which together with the daily yoga practice result in unusual effectiveness. In this environment you learn to rely on yourself, which makes for candidness that breaks through all manners and masks, behind which you might otherwise hide and forget yourself.

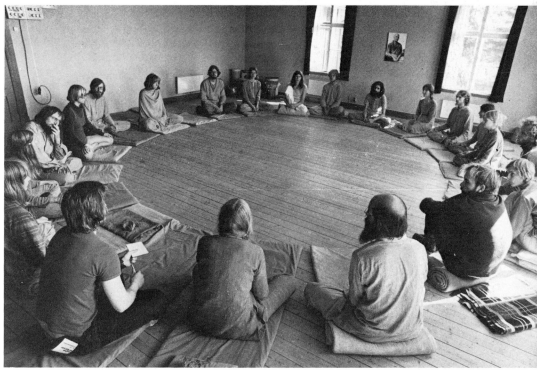

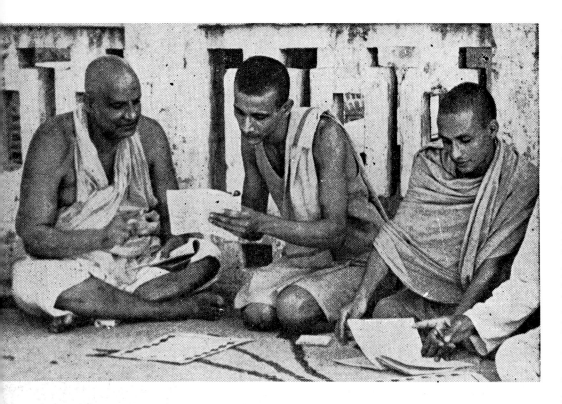

Daily life is the starting point, the situation in which you naturally find yourself, but the workshop is also a yogic laboratory situation: it mirrors us, keeps us alert and sturdy, enables us to see how we might work together with a common goal. This goal is the individual's ability to conquer basic problems both in him or herself and in relation to society, to find one's own way of self-expression.

When you don't know the country,
you ask someone who does!
Led by the knowledgeable guide
he goes forward.
This is truly the happy fruit
of good instruction;
He finds the Way that leads directly forward.
(Rig Veda)

The Teacher

Often we hear the word *guru*, which means "one who disperses the darkness of ignorance".

To experience real alertness in every day and in meditation and to make sure that the methods are working properly, it is necessary to follow the instructions carefully and precisely.

The teacher is the one who transmits his knowledge in such a way that instead of an empty lesson learned by rote, it becomes an experience.

The aspirant must be freed from fear of the unknown during his or her training, so that insight can come without hindrance. Later, when alone, the aspirant can look fear and difficulties in the eye whenever they arise.

The teacher-aspirant relationship is a mutual relationship. It is the task of the aspirant to be open to the teacher, but he or she must also show interest in the task and continue on the path once it is chosen. In this way the teacher is inspired - and without inspiration, there is no teacher.

The Swami

Swami means to be oneself, to reveal one's attitude to life. The swami's goal is to live without fear and to penetrate to the core of life without becoming attached to any special interests; only the innermost and therefore the broadest human interests are the aim. Petty personal ideas, religion that has become a conceited defence, politics, the social norms: the swami feels no obligation towards these things, but chooses to confront and deal with human weakness and doubt, and win human strength. This is **his/her** indispensable function in society.

Meditation and working with yourself can be compared with the work of an artist: it can never be bound or confined in a rigid system. The capacity of this science to remain alive therefore depends on whether it can adapt to the change of different epochs and cultural norms, and in any age be able to enrich the new human being: the human being of today.

The different techniques work through precise learning. However, the experience of being is passed on to those who are open and capable of receiving it from another human being - one who has matured into it. Such a person need not make him/herself known except to those who truly want the experience and who are able to meet themselves straightforwardly.

To work with yourself is of course something which you do not complete in one day. It is a process that takes many years during which the person is opened gradually to a greater capacity to participate in life. From the moment you start, something happens - you don't have to be impatient or bored.

Part Two
The Body, Breathing and Energy

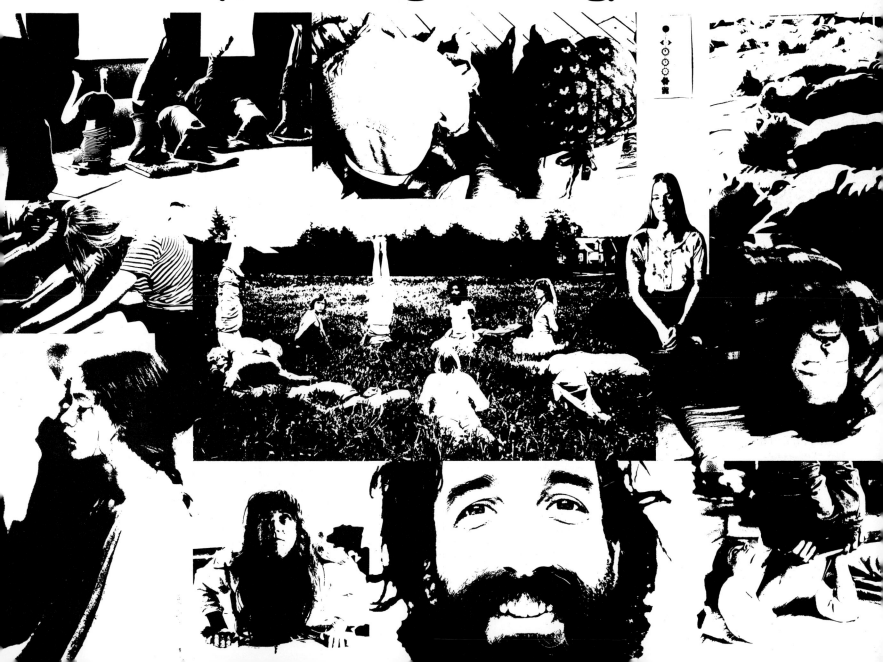

Chapter 6

How to use a Yoga Programme

Introduction

This chapter is about the use of yoga poses. These poses or postures have been arranged into sequences, which we will call programmes.

A programme can be used as a daily practice, or whenever you need it. It can be done in the morning, or, if the morning is not convenient, then in the afternoon between the end of work and the evening meal. Thus it forms a prelude to the whole day or to your free time in the evening.

You can change as you wish between the different programmes we have chosen in this chapter, once you have mastered them. For a while you may be more interested in one programme than the others and go into it in more depth, or you may change between the programmes according to your needs and inclinations.

A programme takes about one hour to complete, counting breathing exercises and a little relaxation. If an hour is too much, choose some of the exercises from these programmes and alternate them so that over a period of days you go through the whole programme and learn it all.

One thing you should know: an effective yoga programme increases your feeling of well being, so it is not a question of wasting time. The time spent doing the exercises becomes a stimulating experience. You may be refreshed after taking a walk, but the effect of a yoga programme reaches deep and lasts long - and apart from a state of increased well being, you experience yourself.

You will make up for time spent many times over with greater alertness and more energy. But don't take my word for it - see for yourself.

How a programme works

Why do we arrange yoga poses in a certain order? Well, the various exercises work differently, so there is a point to starting with certain ones and ending with others.

Some exercises go together in pairs, i.e. pose/counterpose, for example a forward bending and a backward bending exercise, so that the body bends both ways, resulting in harmonious development. The programmes express different temperaments; in some you do a lot of body movement, in others you stay motionless in the different poses, getting a deeper effect.

How to use a programme

1. Lie on your back with your arms at your sides and your feet a little bit apart. This is called "Dead Still". Remain completely motionless all the time.

2. If your mind is busy, give it a while to let go of the thoughts. Then think about what you're going to do next, experience yourself

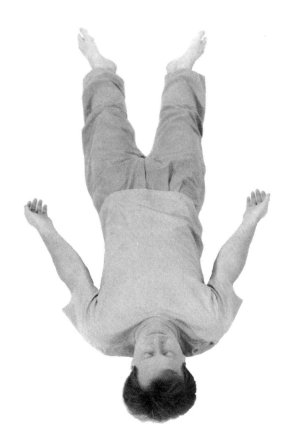

in this situation, picture your body doing the various exercises.

Now find out how it feels when you experience your whole body, the shape of your body - from within, from without. The whole body. Encompass your whole body with your awareness, from head to toe.

Go to your hands and feel them intensely. Just your hands. And after a while, your whole body again. The entire body.

Then watch your breathing. How does the body breathe? Natural breathing. Without influencing it in any way, experience the body breathing. First feel how the body moves. Then feel how air passes in and out of your nostrils.

Become aware of yourself: I am lying here - now.

Prepare yourself to start with the first pose.

3. Do the different poses in their set order. Pay attention to what I say about pausing between different exercises. In some programmes there are few pauses; in others, there are pauses between almost all the exercises. The poses are followed by breathing exercises. **Note:** Always breathe through your nose unless otherwise instructed.

A pause is a period of time during which you experience the effect of the pose settling and the body coming to rest. Remain lying down until just before you get bored, drowsy or restless. At that point go on to the next pose.

A course of exercises can often be divided into: a) warming up, b) getting effects, and c) calming down, when the body and psyche are harmonized. (One of the poses used at the end of some programmes can be called *the union of body and psyche* - the delusion that body, mind and consciousness are separate is dispelled. See the Yoga Attitude p. 79.)

Let us think of yoga as a chance to achieve a greater ability to experience, perceive and feel.

When we go travelling, when we see new things, when we meet with the unexpected, our minds open up and we receive all im-

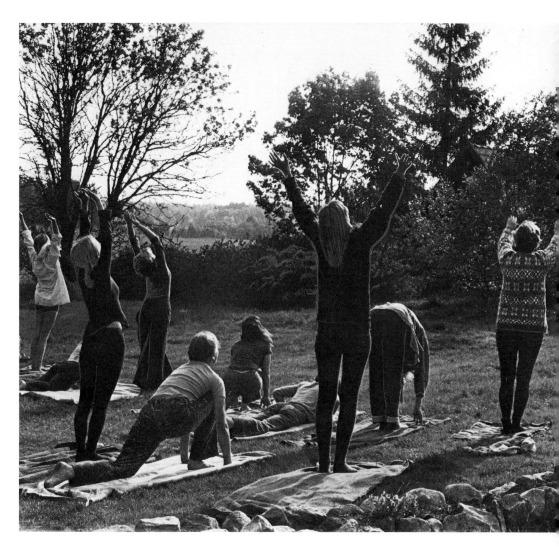

pressions with undiminished strength. When in love, your body is sensitive to the slightest touch - it is new and intense. The ability to experience strongly and freshly all the time; to awaken in the body, to experience its every move, the foot being placed on the ground when it walks, the wind blowing against your skin; to feel how your body tenses when you are overwhelmed or terrified; or to experience what happens in your body when somebody is

making you happy - all these are possible. And you may ask: How do I tackle this? How can I achieve a stronger and more robust relationship with my body? How can I live fully in the body? How can I become one with it?

Start with the first or second programme and feel how you move following the instructions, see yourself sit or lie in the different poses and experience your breathing.

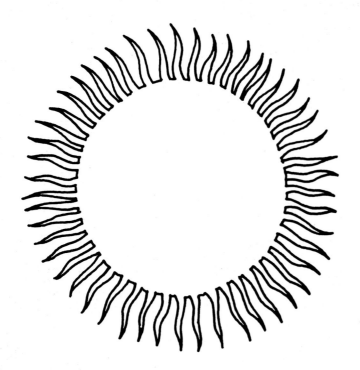

Sun I Greet You

First a programme that can be used at any time by anyone. *Sun I Greet You* is a complete cycle, and some people find this is enough for their daily yoga practice. It fully exercises the body, giving it an energy and well being that is needed throughout the day.

The sequence consists of 2 x 12 poses linked together in a long, flowing motion. 12 poses, each which in its way keeps the body fit - affecting the organs and stretching muscles and tendons; and removing superfluous fat. 12 different ways to work on the spine to release tension throughout the body. The central nervous system is located in the spinal cord and networks throughout the body: affect the spine and you affect the whole body. 12 movements which pump blood through the blood vessels, thus

ensuring that your circulation is kept strong and healthy. The breath is also involved.

In this programme you experience how the inhalation is simultaneous with the backward bending movement. And when you lean forward you exhale. This relationship between body and breath provides the foundation for the most harmonic performance of the exercise.

The breath follows the movement fully. When the inhalation begins, the movement begins. The inhalation is completed when the body leans as far back as it can. Hold it there for a moment. Then begin to exhale and lean forward into the next pose.

2 x 5 full breaths follow the body's movements to give harmony and balance to your breathing and thus to both mind and body.

4 ways to use "Sun, I greet you"

a. Learn and practise. The poses are performed slowly, taking great care to match breathing with movement. Hold each pose a while. Do it all as correctly as possible, but relaxed: Are your feet properly placed? And your hands? Is your back sufficiently stretched? Is the pose tight?

Do a few rounds at first and then choose a number up to a maximum of twelve double rounds. First do the round without thinking about your breathing, then include it when you have mastered the movements and poses.

b. The poses are done as in **a.** but very quickly and at least six times or more so that the body loses its reluctance to move. Let your breathing be strong and noisy - through your nostrils.

c. The poses are performed as in **a.** with the addition of concentration. After a while when you can do the poses automatically and without difficulty, you will be able to concentrate on the body's chakras, focusing in each pose on the corresponding chakra. (When you have reached this stage, see first chapter 8 on the chakras.)

d. If you wish to benefit fully from "Sun, I greet you", you should **either** experience a mantra in each pose, so that the vibration set up by the mantra can affect your mind and body. There is a mantra for each pose, which can also be thought of as a symbolic homage to the sun. **Or,** you can do twelve rounds and before each round of 12 poses you can chant the corresponding mantra. These mantra give you twelve different experiences of the sun rising at dawn every day throughout the year.

If you have a high fever caused by toxic substances in your body, refrain from using this particular programme until the fever has subsided.

The 12 poses follow here:

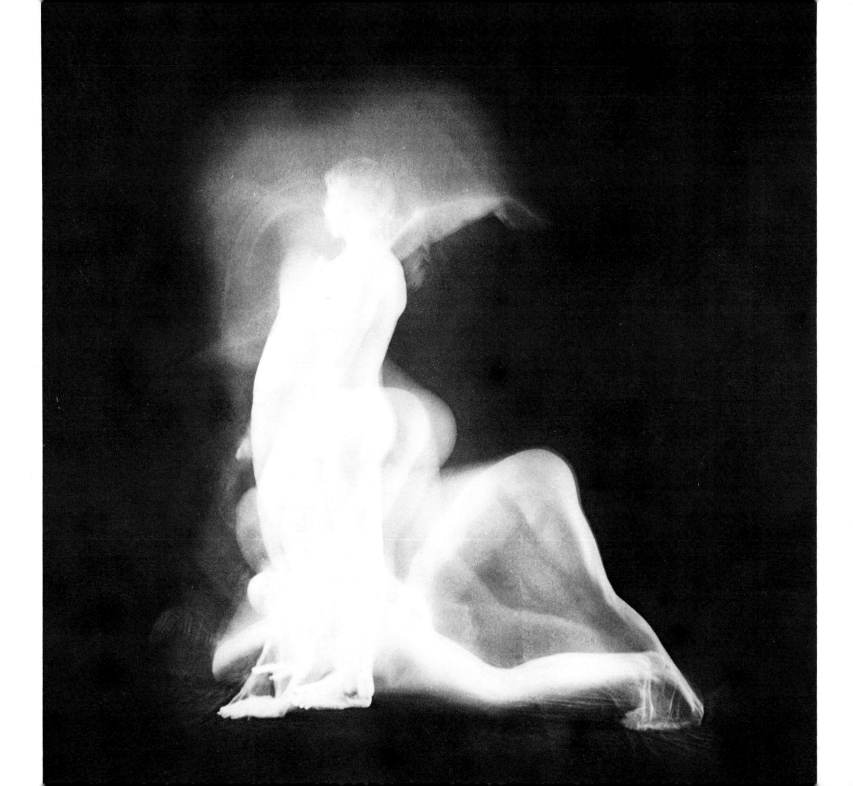

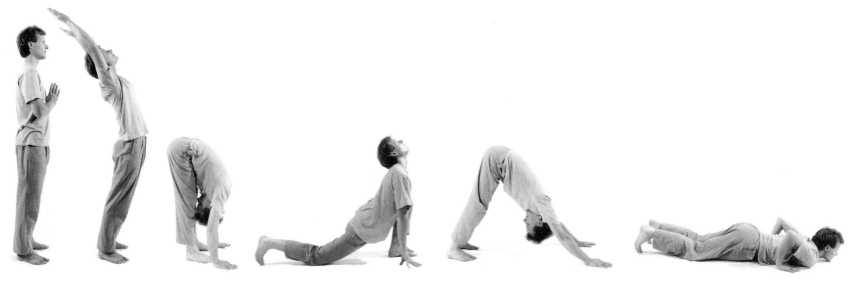

1 ...... inhale .... 2 ..... exhale .... 3 .... inhale deeply .... 4 .... exhale deeply .... 5 .... hold your breath .... 6 ....

1. Greeting

Stand up straight with your feet together. Hold your hands, palms together, in front of your chest. Relax your whole body, prepare yourself to do the round. At a later stage, if you wish to concentrate on the corresponding chakra, feel Anahata Chakra near the heart. If you wish to use a mantra, mentally hear or say aloud: (a) *OM Hram* (short vowel) or (b) *OM Mitraya Namaha* (*OM* - friend to all, I greet you). This is the starting point, creating a state of rest in the body and mind. Inhale while you raise your arms and stretch them back over your head.

2. Stretching the body

Your arms are stretched up backwards, slightly parted, your back slightly arched. Experience openness and receptivity in your body, stretching in the sun's light. Concentrate on Vishuddhi Chakra at the throat. The mantra is *OM Hrim* or *OM Ravaye Namaha* (*OM* - radiant one, I greet you). And now... breathe out while you bend forward

and touch the floor next to your feet, if possible. Your legs are kept straight. Your head should hang down relaxed.

3. Hands by your feet

In this pose, knees straight, if possible touch your knees with your head. And empty your lungs completely by pulling your stomach up. Concentrate on Swadhisthana Chakra behind the sex organs at the base of the spine. The mantra is *OM Hroom* or *OM Suryaya Namaha* (*OM* - you who inspire me to act, I greet you). Inhale as you move one leg back and let that knee touch the floor, while your hands and the other foot stay put. Your forward leg is bent in the motion.

4. The Equestrian pose

Extend your leg as far back as possible. Now your hands, the foot, and the toes and knee of the leg you moved back should all touch the floor. Lean your head back and look up towards the eyebrow centre. The concentration

is on Ajna Chakra in the middle of the head, in a straight line behind the eyebrow centre. The mantra: *OM Hraim* or *OM Bhanave Namaha* (*OM* - you who illumine, I greet you).

When you exhale, move the forward leg back beside the other leg, push your buttocks up, draw your head down between your shoulders until arms, legs and body form a triangle with the floor.

5. The Mountain pose

Empty your lungs. Keep your heels on the floor. Concentrate on Muladhara Chakra, the root chakra just above the perineum. The mantra is *OM Hraum* or *OM Khagaya Namaha* (*OM* - you who move through space, I greet you). After exhaling, hold your breath, lower your body until only your chin, chest, knees, feet and hands touch the floor.

6. Greeting in 8 parts

See that your buttocks, thighs and abdomen are off the floor, and keep your lungs empty

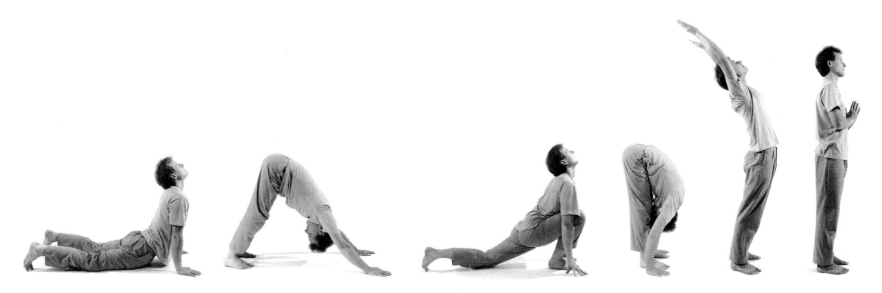

inhale deeply .... 7 .... exhale deeply .... 8 .... inhale deeply .... 9 ...,.............. exhale all the way ... 10 deep inhalation . 11 relaxed exhalation 12

while you stay in this pose. The concentration is on Manipura Chakra behind the navel. The mantra: *OM Hrah* or *OM Pushne Namaha* (*OM* - you who give strength, I greet you). When you have to breathe again, inhale while bending your upper torso and head backwards, until your arms are straight. This is a variation of the classic...

7. Cobra pose

The concentration is on Vishuddhi Chakra at the throat. The mantra is *OM Hram* or *OM Hiranya Garbhaya Namaha* (*OM* - symbol of the golden shape of the universe, I greet you). Now raise your buttocks again until you form a triangle with the floor - as you exhale.

8. The Mountain pose

Like Pose 5. The mantra is *OM Hrim* or *OM Marichaye Namaha* (*OM* - lord of the dawn, I greet you). Move one leg forward until that foot rests on the floor between your hands, while you inhale.

9. The Equestrian pose

Same as 4. Focus on the eyebrow centre.

The mantra is: *OM Hroom* or *OM Savitre Namaha* (*OM* - you who enliven all things, I greet you).

Exhale and move the rear foot forward to the foot between your hands, which still touch the floor. Your legs are straight.

10. Hands by your feet

Same as 3.

The mantra is: *OM Hraim* or *OM Arkaya Namaha* (*OM* - you who deserve all homage, I greet you).

While inhaling deeply, rise and stretch your arms back over your head.

11. Stretching the body

Same as 2. The mantra is: *OM Hraum* or *OM Adityaya Namaha* (*OM* - you who bear the eternal cosmic mother's name, I greet you).

Bring your arms down, palms together, in front of your chest during a relaxed exhalation.

12. Greeting

Like 1. Mantra: *OM Hrah* or *OM Bhaskaraya Namaha* (*OM* - you who lead us to inner enlightenment, I greet you).

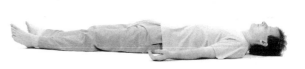

Rest at least three minutes in the "Dead Still".

One complete round of "Sun, I greet you" consists of **two** sequences of the twelve poses. In the first sequence move your left leg back in pose 4 and forward in pose 9. In the second sequence, move the right leg back in 4 and forward in 9. Two times twelve poses form one round - one flowing, continuous course of twenty-four poses.

31

This is a series of easy exercises that everyone can do without difficulty. They are very effective and swiftly give an astonishing feeling of wellbeing.

They are the poses that basically release wind from the intestines and also release tensions and free joints and muscles of stiffness and toxins. Exercises 1 to 17 are beneficial to people suffering from arthritis.

It is a well-known fact to people who work with physical exercises that body tensions and stiffness are closely connected with suppressed psychological problems. One of the secrets behind the physical yoga is the way it releases tensions that represent these problems in muscles and inner organs, in the nervous system and in irregular breathing. This may account for the wellbeing you get from yoga poses and breathing exercises. It makes you realize how these tensions were robbing you of the urge to develop, to have good ideas and to be something to other people - how tensions confined your energy and maybe even led to disease.

When a tension is released, the body has more energy at its disposal - depression vanishes and inspiration reappears.

When you carry out this programme, do it easily and effortlessly, that is, don't try too hard or take too long over any pose, go through the programme moderately fast. All these poses, including the Alternate Breathing on page 43, should take about an hour. (If you don't have enough time, then select one or two of the sections at a time followed by the breathing exercise and go through the whole programme over a few days.)

Even those who have learned more "advanced" yoga maintain that they benefit from these exercises. Besides the local effect of a particular exercise, the programme is refreshing to your state in general. Through the light and swift touch to all the parts of the body, it awakens you to a more conscious feeling and experience of the whole body.

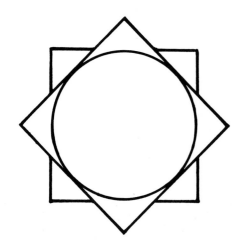

The Small Wind- and Tension-releasing Exercises

A programme for beginners,
for the elderly,
for the ill who are regaining their health,
a programme which has an effect in itself
but which, first of all, is a preparation for
the following exercises in this book.

Section 1
The small tension-release

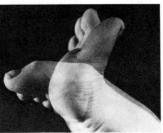

1. Sit with your legs straight out. Bend and stretch your toes. 5-10 times.

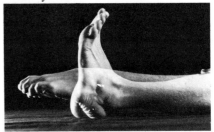

2. Stretch your feet forward and bend them back. 5-10 times.

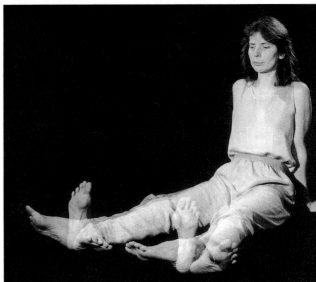

3. Sit with your feet apart, rotate your feet from the ankles. 5-10 times in each direction.

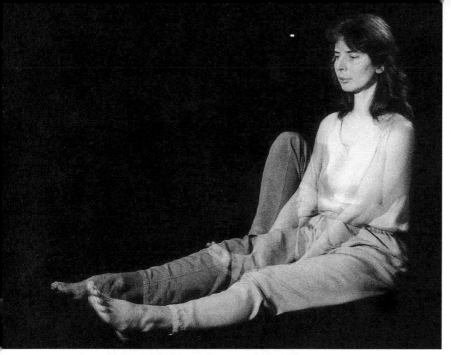

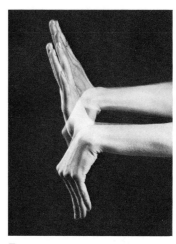

7. With fingers and arms straight, move the hands from the wrists, up and down. 5-10 times.

4. Clasp your hands under your right thigh, and bend the leg so that the heel is as close as possible to your buttocks and bend the foot back with the toes pointing up. Stretch the leg and foot out, without touching the floor. 5-10 times. Change to the left leg. Blood-pumping.

reach keeping your legs straight. Stretch your left arm back and look back at the palm. Then touch your left hand to your right toes, stretching your right arm back. Look back at that hand. Repeat 5-10 times from side to side, gradually increasing the distance between your feet. This exercise makes your spine flexible and releases tensions there.

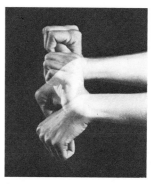

8. Then make fists and move them up and down. 5-10 times.

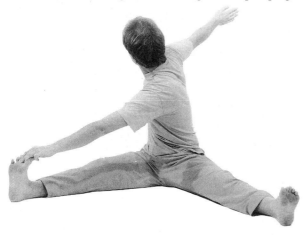

5. Sit with your legs straight out and well apart. Touch your left toes with your right hand, or as far down the left leg as you can

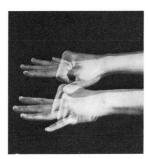

6. Hold your arms out at shoulder level. Spread your fingers and stretch them. Make fists with your thumbs inside your fingers. 5-10 times.

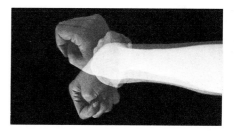

9. Straight arms. Rotate your fists from the wrists. 5-10 times in each direction.
(The other hand can support the arm at the elbow if necessary.)

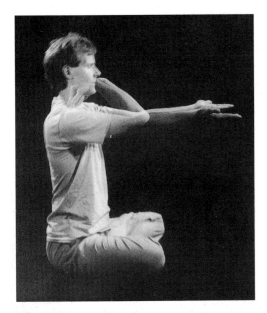

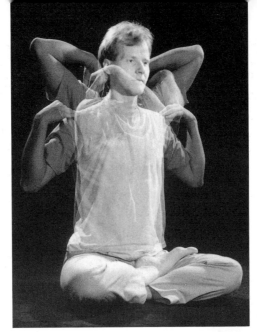

10. Extend your arms forward, shoulder level, palms up. Bend your arms, placing your fingertips on your shoulders. Keep your upper arms horizontal. 5-10 times.

12. Rest your fingertips on your shoulders throughout this exercise. Begin with your upper arms at shoulder level, elbows pointing sidewards. Then rotate your arms, making your elbows meet down in front of your stomach, keep them together as your arms rise up in front of your face and then turn them out to the sides, back and down again in a circular motion. 5-10 times. Repeat the exercise in the opposite direction. This limbers up your shoulders and the upper part of your neck.

14. Rowing

Sit with arms and legs straight in front of you. Move your hands, keeping your arms straight in a vertical circular motion. Lean as far forward and backward as possible and make the circle as wide as you can. 5-10 times in each direction.

Good for digestion and for pregnant women, who should, however, avoid leaning too far back.

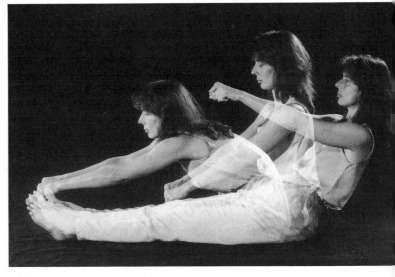

13. Pause

Lie stretched out on your back with your hands at your sides for a while.

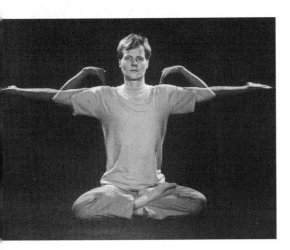

11. Do the same movement, but with your arms out to the sides of your body.

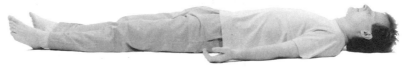

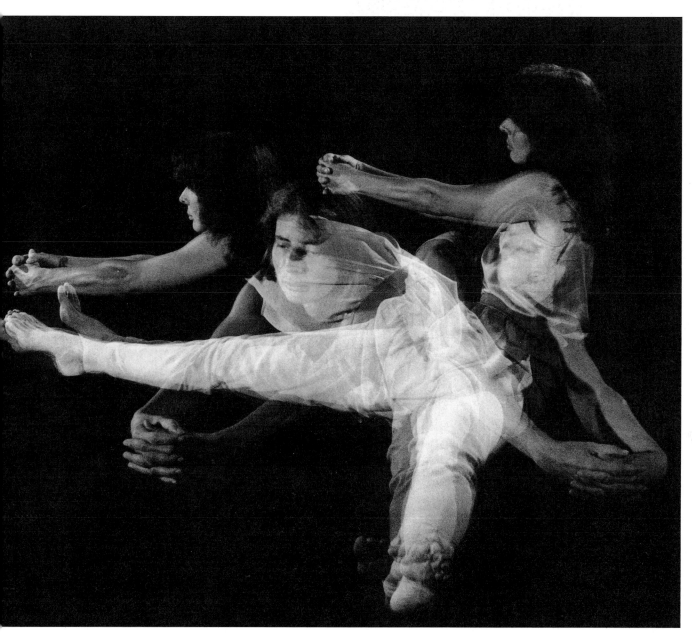

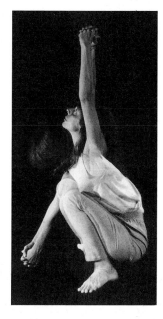

15. The Mill

Sit with straight legs wide apart and your hands clasped. Keep your arms straight and move your hands in a wide circular horizontal motion, letting your upper body follow as far as you can to each side and as far forward and back as possible. 5-10 times in each direction. The same effect as rowing.

16. Chopping

Squat in the so-called *nature pose*. The soles of your feet should be flat on the floor. Make a chopping motion up over your head with straight arms and clasped hands. Good for pregnant women: it develops the breast and affects the milk glands. It also exercises the sacral area and muscles exerted in childbirth.

17. Head Rolling

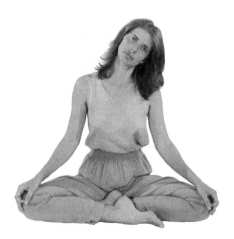

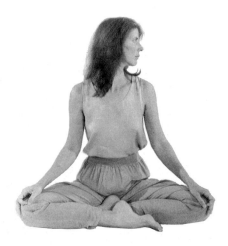

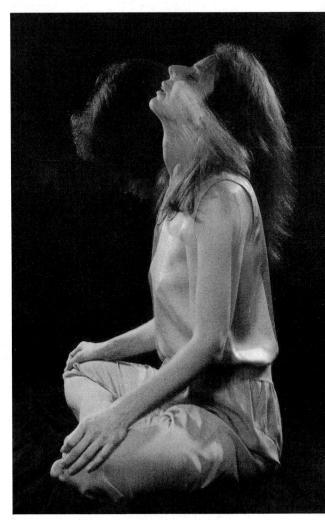

1. Let your head slowly fall all the way to one side, your nose forward, not towards your shoulder. Hang your head like that for a while, then bring it slowly over to the other side and keep it there briefly.
   Repeat this 5-10 times.

2. Turn your head all the way to one side, pause a moment, then turn your head slowly to the other side and pause there.
   Repeat this 5-10 times.

3. Let your head slowly sink down to your chest, let it rest there briefly, totally relaxed, then slowly raise it and rest it there, hanging it back a while. 5-10 times.

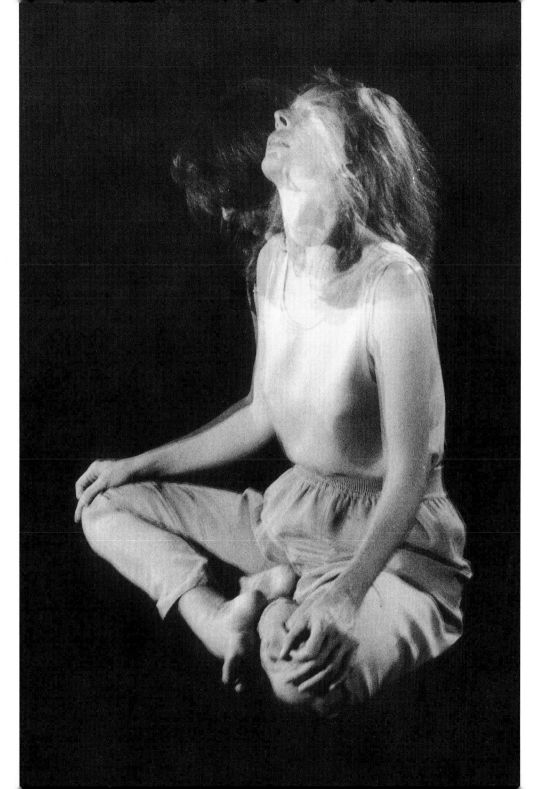

4. Let your head rotate all the way around 5-7 times in each direction. Do it in a very relaxed way and take your time. Feel the position of the head at any one point of the circle.

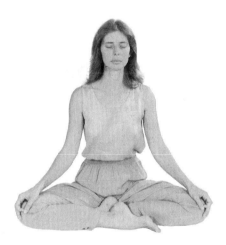

5. Pause immediately after the Head Rolling: sitting relaxed and completely still with your head upright and your eyes closed.

The Head Rolling should not be done if there is dizziness, migraine or high blood pressure.

Section 2

Pre-meditation poses

These exercises make the legs flexible, and strengthen the nerves and the circulation.

They are used to remedy various leg problems, but are best known as pre-meditation poses.

It is fine to start meditating even if you can't sit in a meditation pose, e.g. the Lotus pose. You can start by sitting in a straight-backed chair or on the floor with your back against the wall and your legs straight out in front of you.

In really deep meditation, however, it is important for the body to stay completely motionless for longer periods of time without becoming tired. It is important for the body to conserve and evenly distribute the energy that it acquires through meditation. For this, the pyramid form of the body sitting in a true meditation pose with a straight spine is absolutely essential.

The pre-meditation poses slowly and harmoniously train the body to be able to sit for longer periods of time in these poses. If you want to sit in a meditation pose, practise these exercises for about ten minutes a day.

One mistake that beginners make is to do them too resolutely - if you want to be able to sit in a meditation pose, first of all change your attitude. You may think of meditation as something special and difficult that one achieves only through strenuous efforts. Yet, the state of meditation is reached by letting go and so, to a certain extent, are the meditation poses. Many people find the original poses on page 84 and 85 very natural. And this has nothing to do with the length of your legs or any other physiological reason. This is something everyone can learn and benefit from.

So first of all be aware of your attitude and do not fight your body - work at it in a long-term way, as patiently and as relaxed as possible. "Rome wasn't built in a day!"

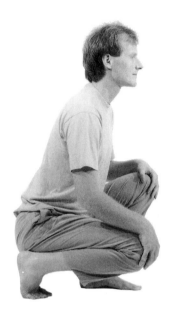

18. The Crow Walk

Squat with your hands on your knees. Walk around the room like that, putting your heels down on the floor first. Walk on the flat sole.

Go all the way down in the pose with each step. The exercise makes your knees flexible and improves the blood circulation in the legs.

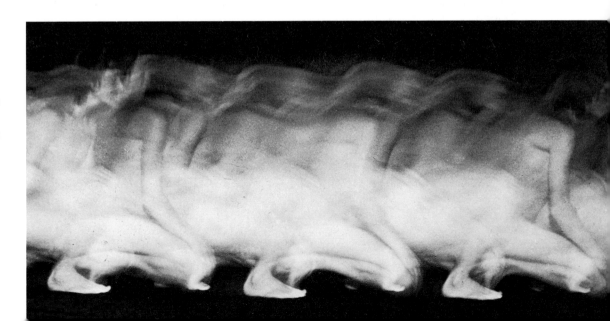

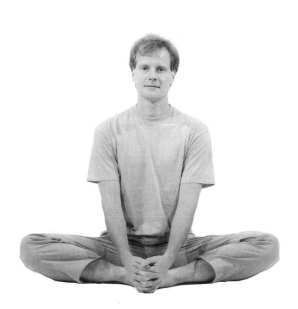

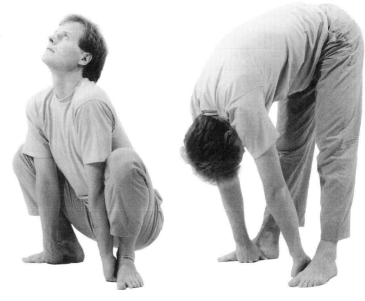

19. The Butterfly

Sit with the soles of your feet together, clasp your hands around them, pull your feet as close to your body as you can and gently pump your legs up and down.

This exercise makes your legs supple and relaxes your lower abdomen, so it is very useful for pregnant women.

Variation: Rock your legs and the lower body from side to side without moving your upper body.

20. The Pump

Squat down. Place your arms between your knees, slipping your palms in under the arches of your feet. Exhale and rise until your legs are straight, letting your head hang down.

Then inhale again as you squat and look up.

Repeat the exercise 5-10 times. This relieves the back, releases blocks and awakens psychic energy.

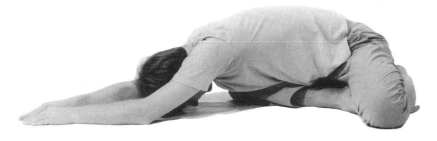

21. The Animals' Relaxation pose

Sit on the floor with one leg bent, so that the heel presses against your groin and the sole of that foot rests against the other thigh. Bend the other leg back so that the heel rests tightly against your buttocks. Rest your hands on the forward leg. Inhale and raise your arms straight over your head; exhale, lowering your arms and upper torso forward over the forward knee until your arms and head rest on the floor. Relax your whole body. Stay in that pose for a while, breathing normally. Then inhale, lifting your torso and arms straight up over your head. Exhale and rest your hands on your knee. Repeat the exercise, changing leg positions.

Section 3

This programme of exercises counteracts difficulties in your digestive tract and releases gas and toxins from the intestines.

Some of the exercises, like the Lion and the Boat, also release deeper-seated physical tensions. These exercises go further than those in Section 1; but anyone can do them without great difficulty or previous knowledge. Through these exercises you can promote physical well being and relaxation.

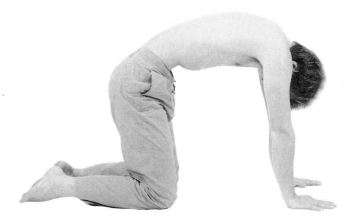

23. The Cat

Get down on all fours. Exhale, raise your back up, hang your head between your shoulders. On inhalation arch your back, while raising your head up and back.

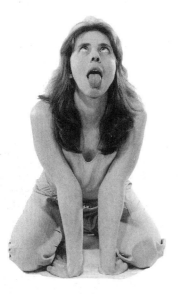

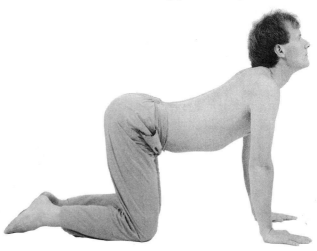

22. The Lion

Sit in the Diamond pose (see p. 58) with your knees apart. Place your hands between your knees, fingers pointing in towards the body. Let your head hang forward. Inhale and raise your head, concentrate on your eyebrow centre, stick out your tongue as far towards your chin as you can and make a deep, forceful sound like a lion roaring as you exhale, or like the "aaah" you make for the doctor. Then relax, letting your head fall forward. Repeat 5-10 times.

Good for the voice, the nose and the throat. Relieves ear troubles. The Lion is used with The Boat to remedy stuttering.

Variation: The Dog.
Sit in the same pose as for the Lion. Stretch out your tongue and pant like an over-heated dog, with short, shallow and fast breaths. Good for the diaphragm and the basis for natural abdominal breathing.

A more advanced variation: Empty your lungs and raise your back, then pull your diaphragm up and in, pull in your anal muscles; hold as long as you can. Then relax your anal muscles and your abdomen and arch your back while inhaling. The Cat can be repeated 3-5-10 times. It is good for the back and the small of the back and is highly recommended for pregnant women, who should keep their legs apart and should not pull in the stomach.

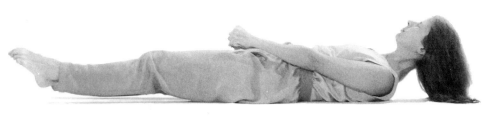

24. The Boat

Variation 1:

Lie on your back with your arms extended a couple of inches over your thighs. Make fists. Inhale, hold your breath and lift your legs and head a few inches off the floor, so that your head and toes are level. Clench your teeth, tense your whole body; hold the pose as long as possible. Then relax completely so that you thud down on the floor. Repeat 3-5 times.

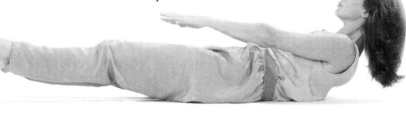

Variation 2:

Stretch out your hands, hold your breath in the pose but don't clench your teeth, then slowly relax your body.

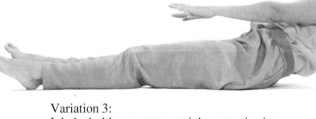

Variation 3:

Inhale, hold your arms straight out, raise just the upper torso.

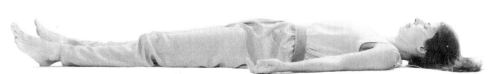

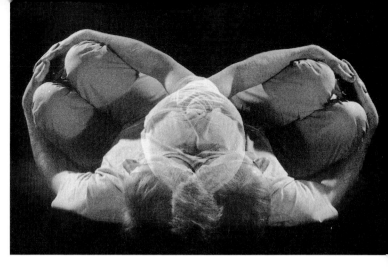

25. Rock and Roll

Lie on your back with bent knees and hands clasped around your knees. Rock from side to side so that the small of the back is massaged. Let your head and shoulders roll on the floor.

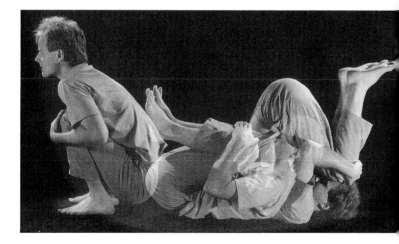

Roll back and forth with your hands around your knees. Each time roll up so that you squat on the soles of your feet with your buttocks off the floor, then roll backward up on the shoulders and back, with the head bent forward against the knees.

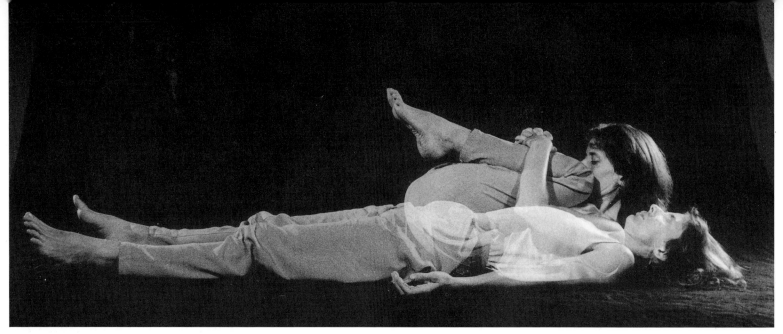

26. Wind-releasing pose

Lie on your back. Inhale, bend your right leg, hands clasped around that knee and gently press the thigh softly against the stomach.

Then exhale while raising your head and let your nose touch your knee. With empty lungs, lower your head and leg again.

Inhale while bending the left leg and repeat the exercise; then repeat with both legs together.

This forms one round. Repeat 4-5 rounds.

The exercise releases gas in the intestines.

27. The Hare

Sit in the Diamond pose. Hold your left wrist behind your back. Lean forward and rest your forehead on the floor. Breathe normally. Concentrate from the navel area to a point in your spine behind your navel, the *Manipura Chakra*. Remain in this pose for at least three minutes, preferably longer. Then sit up with your eyes closed and relax completely. Sit absolutely still for a while, experiencing your body from within. Let your consciousness fill your entire body. This has a calming effect on over-excitement, anger, anxiety and depression.

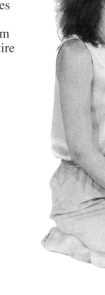

Breathing I

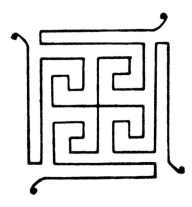

1. Spontaneous Breathing

This is a breathing, relaxation and meditation exercise. Start by lying on your back with your hands at your sides:

Experience your whole body,
the whole body at once,
feel how motionless it is -
concentrate a long time on the motionlessness.

Then begin to experience that
this motionless body is alive, it is breathing;
let it breathe
freely,
avoid slowing down
or speeding up your breathing,
avoid controlling it,
breathe freely,
spontaneously -
go on
go on
as long as possible -
ten minutes - fifteen minutes - half an hour.

After a while
make sure you are breathing with the stomach.
Otherwise use your will a little,
but avoid disturbing
the free rhythm of your breath,
feel -
that you breathe with the stomach;

let your stomach expand
as you inhale,
and let the rest follow;
let your stomach sink down and relax
when you exhale;
do not bother about your mind;
breathe freely and spontaneously
with your attention on
your stomach,
go on -
now notice how your stomach
rises and falls
with natural breathing,
go on -

Use this exercise as often and as long as
you like
any time -
but preferably at regular
times.

2. Alternate Breathing

Sit with your back straight in as harmonious a pose as possible (naturally a meditation pose is best, see pages 84-5). Use your right hand in this exercise: the thumb and ring finger are used to close your nostrils, the index and

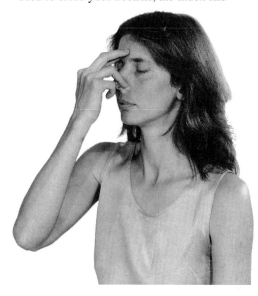

second fingers rest on your forehead.

Close your right nostril with your thumb and inhale slowly and soundlessly through your left nostril, then shut the left with your ring finger and open your right nostril by releasing your thumb.

Exhale as slowly, soundlessly and thoroughly as possible, through your right nostril. Then inhale through the right nostril, shut it with your thumb, open the left nostril and exhale as slowly, soundlessly and completely as you can.

This is one round: at first do a sequence of five rounds and when you have mastered this quite well, slowly raise the number to eleven, then to sixteen, and finally if you wish to twenty-two rounds. Do not go beyond this number. This large number of rounds only applies to this first variation. In the other variations where you hold your breath (pages 49 and 81), you should do no more than five rounds.

Instructions for Breathing Exercises

It is important to follow certain rules in doing these exercises:

1. You will get the most out of breathing exercises if you do them regularly - and at the same time every day.
2. They should be done **after** physical exercises and **before** meditation.
3. Never do breathing exercises until three to four hours after a large meal.
4. Make sure you are not sitting in a cold or draughty place, but always exercise in a well ventilated room.
5. Don't do them when you are excited or short of breath.
6. Don't drink cold water right after the exercises.
7. Wait a while, about forty-five minutes, after these exercises, before you eat a main meal or take a bath - bathe preferably before the exercises rather than afterwards. Always take it easy for at least twenty minutes after breathing exercises, or continue with a meditation.

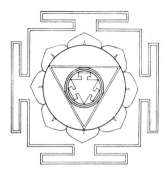

Intermediate Poses

When you have mastered the previous programme (the small wind- and tension-releasing exercises) and have been using it for a while, start this one. You might also alternate them, one day doing one and the next day the other. This programme is an important preparation for the following exercises and programmes: it strengthens the back, making it flexible, and develops balance.

1. The Triangle poses

A.   1. Stand with legs apart, and keep them straight. Extend your arms sideways at shoulder level.

2. As you exhale, twist your body to the right, bend forward and with your left hand touch your right foot, or as far down as you can reach.

3. Look up at your right hand, which points up.

4. As you inhale, straighten up again with your arms at shoulder level.

5. Twist your body to the other side and bend down as you exhale. 5-10 times.

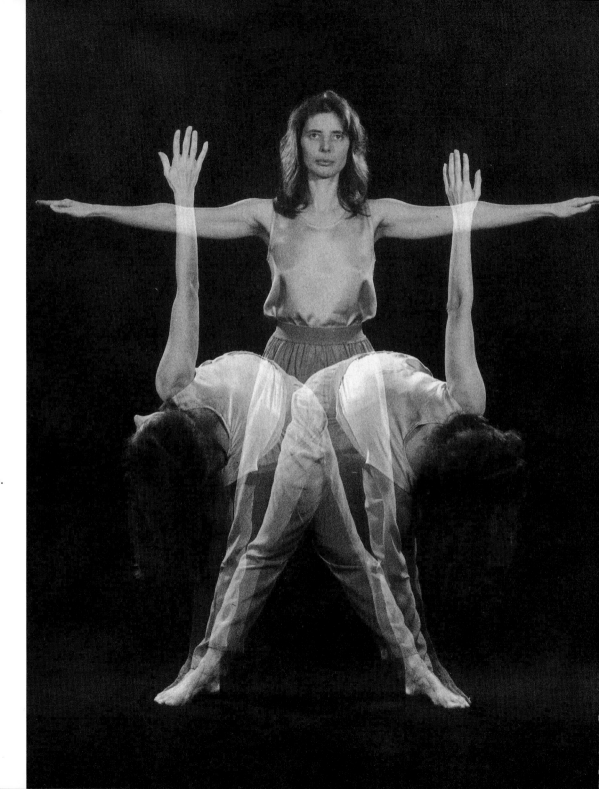

44

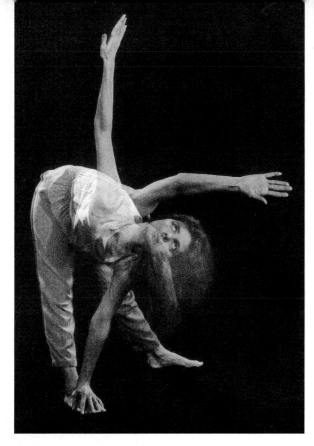

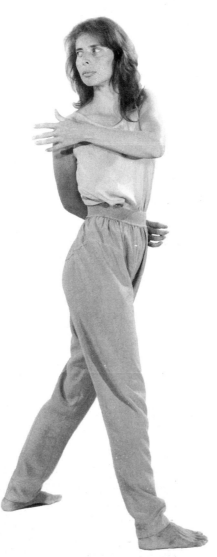

D. 1. Stand with feet apart and arms bent, palms pressed against your body as high up under your arms as possible, the fingers pointing down.

2. Keep your left hand there and let the right hand slide down along the side of your body, while you lean the upper part of your body over to the right as you exhale. Don't lean forward or back, just straight to the side.

3. Inhale as you return to an upright position. Repeat this on the other side. 5-10 times.

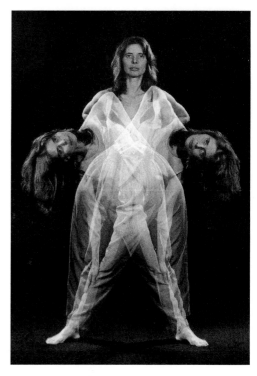

B. Like **A**, but instead of looking up at the raised arm as in step 3, lower and extend that arm horizontally over your head. 5-10 times.

C. 1. Stand with your feet apart and arms hanging at your sides.

2. Start swinging your arms from side to side by twisting your body. When you twist to the right, look as far back as you can over your right shoulder and then to the left.

3. Now swing so far that your left hand ends on your right shoulder and the right hand, drawn behind your back, touches your waist round on the left side, and vice versa. This movement should be so loose that your relaxed arms swing out from the body. 10-20 times.

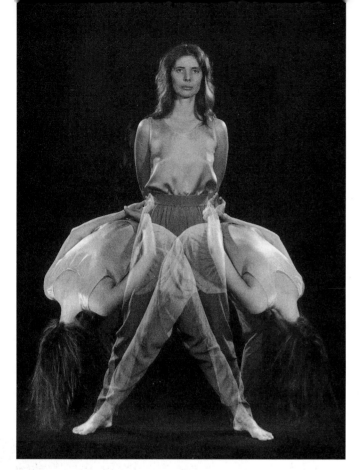

2. Shoulder pose

1. Lie on your back and bend your knees so that the soles of your feet rest on the floor close to your buttocks.

2. Grasp your ankles.

3. Inhale and push your body up so that the weight rests on your shoulders and feet. Relax your neck. Stay in the pose as long as you can hold your breath.

The Shoulder pose is useful in pregnancy, especially after childbirth, since it prevents a displaced uterus and strengthens the sex organs; good if you have a tendency to miscarry. The pose can be used to get slipped

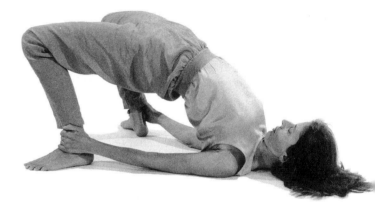

E. 1. Stand with feet apart. Keep your hands behind you, one hand clasping the other wrist.

2. Exhale as you turn a little to the right, bend your right knee slightly and lower your nose towards your knee.

3. Come up again to a straight position as you inhale. Repeat 5-10 times.

F. Like **E** with feet further apart. Now bring your nose as close to your feet as possible.

The Triangle poses are specially good for the spine, which is turned, stretched and bent. The spinal cord is very important to the yogi and must be kept in absolutely top condition. It is the location of the central nervous system and where the yogi works with

energy: Prana and the Kundalini.

Good for nervous depressions. Pose **C** also affects the bowels and aids peristalsis. It stimulates the appetite.

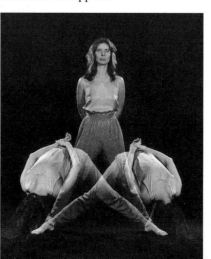

discs into place. It stretches and massages the intestines and the inner abdominal organs. It is good for stooped posture and back pains.

3. The Clown

Make sure you have a soft support for the crown of your head.

1. Rest on your hands and knees.

2. Bend your arms and place your head on the floor. Your lower arms should be vertical.

3. Extend your legs so that your body makes an angle (rest weight on head, toes and hands).

4. Move your legs by rising up on your toes until your knees touch your elbows.

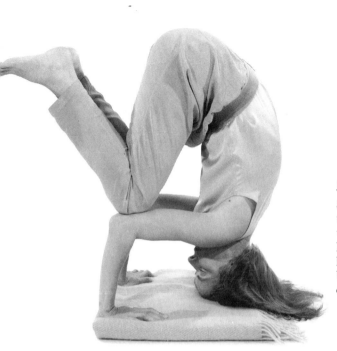

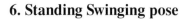

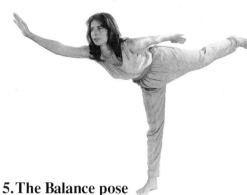

5. Rest your knees on your elbows and lift your feet off the floor, your head and hands remain on the floor. Hold the pose for 1-2 minutes, eventually extending it to 5 minutes.

The Clown may be used instead of or as a preparation for the Headstand which is the most important yoga pose, as it increases the blood supply to the head, relieves the heart, and gives calmness and clarity.

4. The Palm

The opposite of the Clown.

Stand with your arms stretched over your head, hands clasped, palms up. Inhale, rise up on your toes. Balance for a while, looking up at the hands and hold your breath. Then exhale and come down again onto the soles of your feet, lower your arms and stand for a while relaxed, with your arms at your sides.

Variation: Walk around on your toes in this pose. Counteracts constipation: drink some lukewarm water, perhaps with a little salt in it and then do the exercise.

5. The Balance pose

Stand with your feet together. Inhale deeply while raising your right arm. Lean forward while exhaling, so that your torso becomes horizontal, extending your right arm out horizontally over your head, and your left leg back horizontally. You are now balancing on one leg. Breathe normally while in this pose.

Repeat the exercise on the other leg.

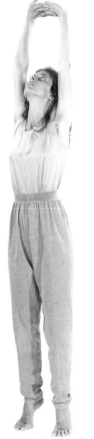

6. Standing Swinging pose

1. Stand with your legs slightly apart. Raise your arms with loose wrists up over your head, while you inhale.

2. Exhale as you let your whole upper body fall forward relaxed.

3. Swing forward to the horizontal position as you inhale and then back between your legs as you exhale, your head, arms and torso relaxed and loose. Keep swinging fast for 20 breaths - forward inhaling, back exhaling.

4. Stop swinging; raise your arms over your head as you inhale.

5. Exhale, lowering your arms, and stand still until your body has come to rest. Then repeat the exercise.

Variation: Exhale, hold your breath and swing forward and back with your whole upper body, neck and arms totally relaxed, for as long as you can.

The Standing Swinging pose should not be done in cases of dizziness, migraine or high blood pressure. It eliminates fatigue, tones your thighs and back muscles, reduces fat, is good for pregnant women and as a preparation for breathing exercises.

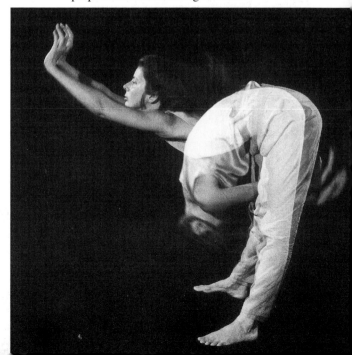

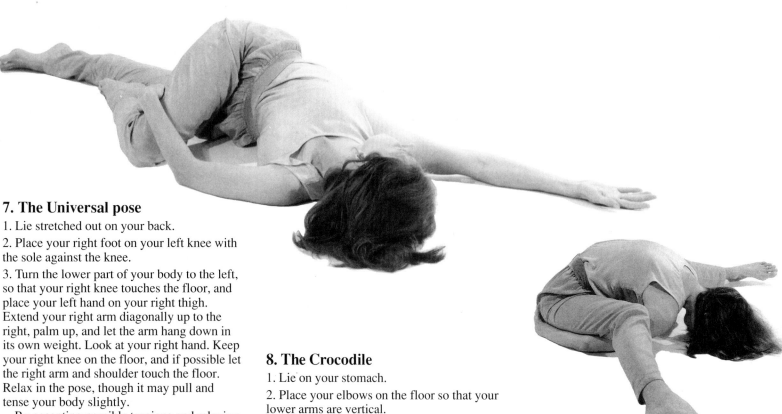

7. The Universal pose

1. Lie stretched out on your back.

2. Place your right foot on your left knee with the sole against the knee.

3. Turn the lower part of your body to the left, so that your right knee touches the floor, and place your left hand on your right thigh. Extend your right arm diagonally up to the right, palm up, and let the arm hang down in its own weight. Look at your right hand. Keep your right knee on the floor, and if possible let the right arm and shoulder touch the floor. Relax in the pose, though it may pull and tense your body slightly.

By accepting possible tensions and relaxing more and more with each breath you will gradually become calm in this pose. Stay there at least a minute and then repeat it on the other side. When you get used to the pose you can stay in it from 5 to 10 minutes to get a deeper effect.

The whole body, particularly the spine, is turned in a spiral; the Universal pose is said to stretch the greatest number of muscles in the body at once.

Relieves disc injuries and sciatica.

8. The Crocodile

1. Lie on your stomach.

2. Place your elbows on the floor so that your lower arms are vertical.

3. Rest your chin in your hands.

Also watch your breathing in this pose and notice how your stomach presses against the floor with each breath.

This is used for resting the back after meditation and gives relief from disc injuries.

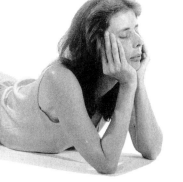

9. The Tortoise

1. Sit on the floor with your legs apart. Bend your legs and torso forward so that you can put one arm under each thigh and knee joint (one at a time). Extend your arms fully so they reach around behind your thighs.

2. Clasp your hands behind your buttocks, palms outward, or get them as close together as you can.

3. Straighten your legs as much as possible, and gradually lower your forehead to the floor. Hold this pose, preferably for five minutes or as long as you can. Exhale while you lean forward, then breathe normally.

The Tortoise has a strong calming effect, it strengthens the mind against disturbances and concludes the programme harmoniously, just as the Hare did in the previous programme.

Breathing II

Now we will proceed to explore further how breathing affects the body and mind and how they can be influenced. The rules which were given in Breathing I naturally apply throughout the book; the longer you do these exercises and the more advanced they are, the more scrupulous you must be about the rules and procedures.

3. The Wave Breath

A. Lie on your back as in exercise **1** (page 43) and feel the stomach breathe for a while.

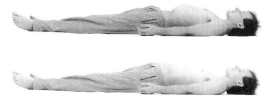

B. Exhale; empty your lungs and roll in the same way with empty lungs.

4. The Blacksmith's Bellows 1

Sit straight with your hands in the same position as in exercise **2** (page 43). Notice which nostril is more open. Close the other nostril with your thumb or ring finger and

through the same nostril. Now change to the other nostril. Repeat the sequence three times with each nostril. This is also used following nose cleaning (page 56) to dry the nose.

The Bellows purifies the blood and provides oxygen - thereby making the brain clearer - and reduces depression. The digestive fire is increased. An effective exercise if you suffer from lung, throat or chest diseases.

5. Alternate Breathing, Variation 2

Do exercise **2** on page 43, but instead of breathing out when you have just inhaled, hold your breath a short while by closing both nostrils with your thumb and ring finger.

Start inhaling with your left nostril, hold your breath, exhale with your right nostril, inhale again with your right, hold your breath and exhale with your left nostril. This forms one sequence. Do **only** five sequences.

When you can manage this without tension, then also hold your breath after exhaling, and inhale with the nostril through which you have just exhaled. (The final version is on page 81.)

6. Psychic Breathing

With your mouth closed, make a whispering, slightly hissing sound in your throat, as if you were fast asleep. Listen to the sound. Make the same sound as you breathe in and out. If the sound is coming from the soft palate, it is incorrect. It should come from the vocal cords further down your throat.

Breathe deeply and slowly, letting the sound extend your breath; pause briefly after inhalation and after exhalation, but make no other effort to change the way you breathe, **only** listen to the sound.

To do this exercise correctly, bend your tongue back so that the tip touches the soft palate. This will increase saliva production and prevent throat irritation.

The Psychic Breathing is relaxing and a suitable preparation for meditation. If you do it properly, you can breathe this way as long as you like. You will experience increased energy.

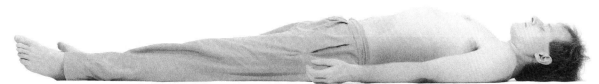

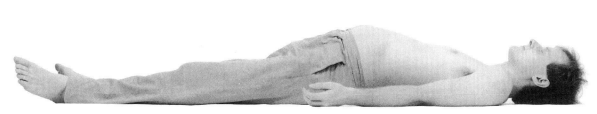

Then inhale by expanding your stomach and hold your breath.
Pull in your stomach and let the bubble of breath roll up into your chest cavity, extending it.
Keep holding your breath, and now let the bubble of air roll down again expanding your stomach, pulling in your chest.
Again let the air expand your chest, and so on, in a fast, even rhythm.
Let the breath bubble roll like a wave, back and forth. Three rounds.

breathe in and out rapidly through the open nostril. As you inhale, extend your stomach and as you exhale pull in your stomach, so that it works like a blacksmith's bellows; thus you breathe with your stomach, not your chest. Do this swiftly and without too much effort, for about twenty breaths, then inhale fully and hold your breath by closing both nostrils. Don't hold it so long that you are straining and don't let the air press too hard in your nose. If you are blocked, hold it long enough to feel both nostrils open. Then exhale slowly

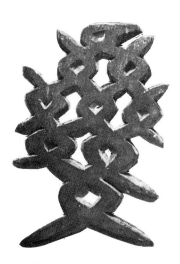

Back Programme

The back programme firstly influences you physically. It works with tensions of the muscles and organs, and more generally with the health of the whole body - the breath is used consciously all the time, through the way you breathe or hold the breath in the different poses.

When you relax in the Best pose at the end of this programme, you also experience a deeper psychic effect, a state of clarity and well being. You feel it in your natural breathing, which is flowing more freely, and all parts of your body are now felt as a living harmonic whole; you and your body are one.

The back is very important in yoga. It is the seat of the central nervous system and of four of the *chakras*. By loosening tensions in the back, many other organs and functions of the body are influenced and the effect of the exercises in this programme is, therefore, not only limited to the back.
Do you normally move your body in certain habitual patterns? Do you use your breath fully? Do you especially use certain muscles while others are left unused? If you do, it will naturally create inertia in some organs and overloading of others. We may see this as an imbalance in the distribution of the energy of the body. The energy does not flow freely, it is blocked. In some parts there is too much tension, experienced as pain in the neck, the back, or the hips. In other parts there is too little tension, experienced as a lack of energy.

The movements, the poses and the breath in this programme bring the body back to its natural carriage. Muscle tensions are loosened, energy blocks are liberated, the spine and its nerves are stretched and massaged, muscles and blood supply are stimulated.

If you have serious problems with the back or the neck you should first train with the Small Wind- and Tension-releasing Exercises (page 32) and the Triangle poses (page 44). After practising these exercises regularly for some time, you achieve more sensitivity and you will be able to feel for yourself how far you can go with the different back strengthening exercises.

The Back Programme is a good preparation for The Classical Programme (page 69).

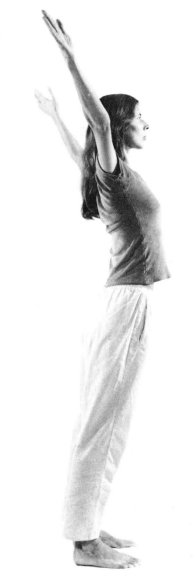

1. Cross pose

1. Stand with the feet together and the wrists crossed in front of the body.
2. Inhale and raise the crossed arms up over the head.
3. Exhale and stretch the arms up at an angle out to the sides. Keep the arms and hands as far back as possible, expand the chest and feel the stretch in the inside of the arms.
4. Raise the arms over the head again on inhalation and cross the wrists.
5. Lower the crossed arms down in front of the body on exhalation. Three rounds.

Loosens up the shoulder area, the chest, and tensions in the upper part of the back.

2. Standing on all Fours

1. Stand with your feet together and the arms alongside the body.

2. Turn your hands upward so that they are at a right angle with the arms, the palms facing downwards.

3. Inhale and stretch the arms up over the head keeping the hands at the same angle. The palms are now facing upwards.

4. Exhale as you bend the upper part of the body and the arms forward until the palms touch the floor. Place the hands so far forward that you can keep the knees straight and place the weight of the body equally on hands and feet. Raise the head and look forward. Stay in the pose as long as you can hold the breath out.

5. Come up again on inhalation raising the arms above the head.

6. Exhale and let the arms and hands hang down loose. Three rounds.

   Stretches and relaxes calf and thigh muscles, makes the hips supple and improves the body posture.

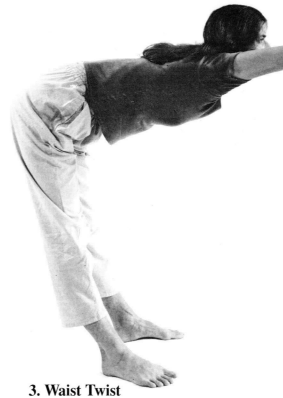

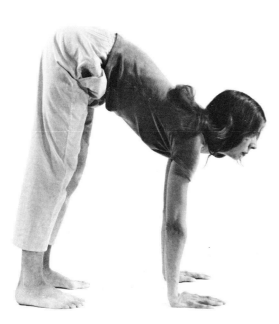

3. Waist Twist

1. Stand with the legs apart and fold the hands in front of the body, palms facing downward.

2. Stretch the arms above the head on inhalation. Now the palms are turned upward.

3. Exhale and bend at the hips so that the small of the back, the back and the arms are pointing forward in a straight horizontal line. Look up at your folded hands.

4. While holding the breath out, twist the upper part of the body and the arms horizontally as far to the right as possible and back to the middle again. Do this three times. Make sure, while you twist the body, that the hands, arms and back are kept straight and horizontal.

5. Come up again on inhalation, moving the arms up above the head.

6. Exhale and lower the arms.

7. Do the exercise once more to the left side.

8. Finally, the third time you do the exercise, twist the body in a full half-circle all the way from the right to the left and back, three times.

   Often, when the back has a faulty carriage it causes tension and pain at the small of the back.

   The Waist Twist makes you aware of the muscles at the small of the back, it strengthens them and makes the whole back supple. The Waist Twist, therefore, is an important exercise in this programme.

4. Double Angle

1. Stand with your feet together.

2. Inhale and fold your hands behind the back.

3. Exhale and let the upper part of the body and the head hang down in front. The hands are resting on the back.

4. Inhale and lower the straight arms till they hang by their own weight away from the back, palms inwards. Keep the knees straight and let the head hang loose. Relax arms and shoulders and feel how the arms slowly lower themselves further. Keep standing in the pose as long as you are able to hold the breath.

5. Exhale, raise the arms to the back again.

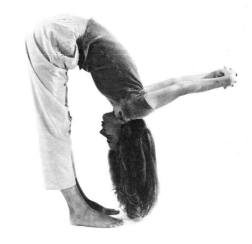

6. Inhale and straighten the body.

7. Exhale, unfold the hands and let the arms hang loosely alongside the body. Three rounds.

The Double Angle increases the blood circulation and loosens tensions in the neck, shoulders and upper part of the back.

5. Quick Plough

For illustration please see page 72.

1. Lie on your back for a moment.

2. Raise the straight legs to a vertical position, then lower them over the head so that the buttocks and the back are lifted off the floor. As soon as the toes touch the floor above the head (or as far as you can without straining yourself), bring the legs back to the original position, lying on your back. Immediately raise them over the head again, till the toes touch the floor - then move them back again to a lying position. Keep moving the legs back and forth this way 8-12 times. Quick, light and easy. Do not hold your breath. Breathe without effort.

3. At the end of these fast movements remain in the Plough pose, with the tips of the toes resting on the floor above the head. Take your time in this position and let your breath calm down completely.

When you first do this, you may bend the knees a little when you have the legs over the head, as this makes it easier for the toes to reach the floor, but aim at keeping them straight.

If you feel that it tenses or stretches you more than is comfortable, for example in the thighs or the calves, then imagine that your breath flows through the tension and loosens it.

Come out of the pose by lowering the legs in a very slow and even movement down towards the floor again.

The Quick Plough harmonizes the nervous system by stretching and massaging the whole spine. It strengthens the abdominal and back muscles.

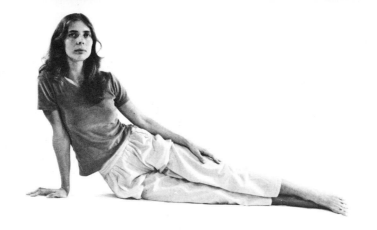

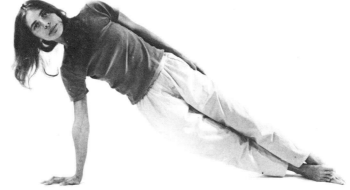

6. The Bridge

A. 1. Lie on your side.

2. Raise the upper part of the body and support it on the arm underneath. The palm is now placed on the floor, the arm is vertical and the upper part of the body is at an angle with the floor. The legs are lying straight on the floor.

3. Inhale and raise the hip from the floor so that the body rests only on one arm and on the side of one foot. The body is now completely straight.

4. Exhale and lower the legs to the floor. Do three rounds to each side.

B. 1. Now sit with the legs stretched in front of you and the hands on the floor behind your back with the fingers pointing backward.

2. Inhale and raise the buttocks 3-4 inches (10 centimetres) above the floor.

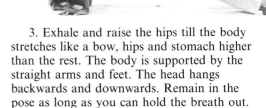

3. Exhale and raise the hips till the body stretches like a bow, hips and stomach higher than the rest. The body is supported by the straight arms and feet. The head hangs backwards and downwards. Remain in the pose as long as you can hold the breath out.

4. Inhale and lower the body, till the buttocks are about 3-4 inches (10 cm.) off the floor.

5. Exhale and lower the body to the floor. Three rounds.

7. Preliminary Backstretch

A. 1. Sit with one leg straight, bend the other, so the sole of the foot is against the thigh of the straight leg and the heel against the groin. The hands are placed on the straight knee.

2. Inhale and stretch the arms up and as far back as possible.

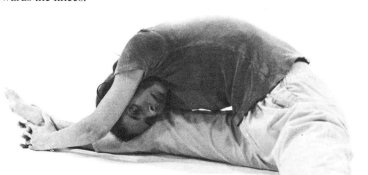

3. Exhale and bend over the straight leg until the upper part of the body is resting on the leg, or is as far forward as possible. Clasp the hands around the foot or ankle. Do not strain yourself here. Let the shoulders hang with the arms slightly bent, and the head hanging down between the arms. Relax the upper part of the body and the stomach.

4. Inhale and sit up again with the arms straight up over the head.

5. Exhale and lower your hands to the knee again. Repeat the exercise with the other leg.

B. is performed like **A**, but now place the foot on top of the thigh.

C. 1. Sit with both legs straight and as far apart as possible. Place the hands on one knee.

2. Inhale and stretch the arms up and back as far as possible.

3. Exhale as you let the upper part of the body hang down over one leg. Clasp the hands, if possible, around the foot. Relax the upper part of the body and the arms and eventually let the head rest against the leg. Keep sitting for a moment and relax in the pose while you hold the breath out.

4. Inhale as you come up again with arms above the head.

5. Exhale as you bend down over the other leg (same as 3).

6. Inhale as you come up again with the arms above the head.

7. Exhale and grab hold around both feet. The upper part of the body is now hanging down between the legs.

8. Inhale as you come up again with arms above the head.

9. Exhale as you lower the arms down towards the knees.

When the arms are stretched up and back, you loosen stiffness in the shoulders, the upper part of the back and the small of the back. By bending forward you stretch and relax the whole back and muscles in the thighs.

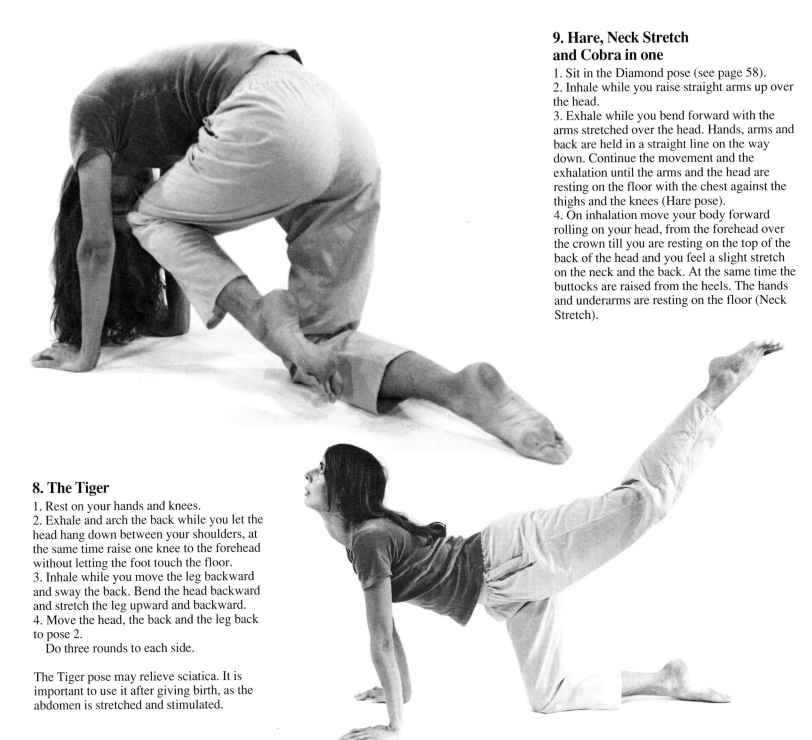

9. Hare, Neck Stretch and Cobra in one

1. Sit in the Diamond pose (see page 58).
2. Inhale while you raise straight arms up over the head.
3. Exhale while you bend forward with the arms stretched over the head. Hands, arms and back are held in a straight line on the way down. Continue the movement and the exhalation until the arms and the head are resting on the floor with the chest against the thighs and the knees (Hare pose).
4. On inhalation move your body forward rolling on your head, from the forehead over the crown till you are resting on the top of the back of the head and you feel a slight stretch on the neck and the back. At the same time the buttocks are raised from the heels. The hands and underarms are resting on the floor (Neck Stretch).

8. The Tiger

1. Rest on your hands and knees.
2. Exhale and arch the back while you let the head hang down between your shoulders, at the same time raise one knee to the forehead without letting the foot touch the floor.
3. Inhale while you move the leg backward and sway the back. Bend the head backward and stretch the leg upward and backward.
4. Move the head, the back and the leg back to pose 2.

   Do three rounds to each side.

The Tiger pose may relieve sciatica. It is important to use it after giving birth, as the abdomen is stretched and stimulated.

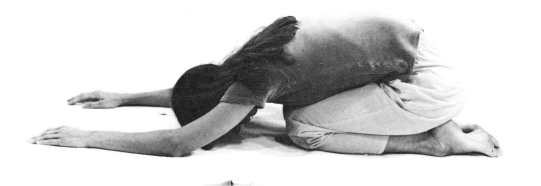

while you exhale until the hands are again resting on the knees as in the initial position (Diamond pose).

The combination of these poses loosens up tensions in several points on the spine.

When the body is hanging relaxed in this variation of the Cobra, the abdominal muscles are stretched and relaxed. (For women, the Cobra strengthens the womb muscles, among other things. If the Cobra is used often it can prevent menstruation pains.)

The movement in and out of the Hare pose stimulates the muscles around the small of the back and takes away stiffness of the hips.

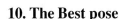

5. Roll back again on exhalation, resuming the Hare pose. Your forehead and arms are now touching the floor.
6. Supporting your weight on the hands and knees, inhale and glide forward close to the floor and up, till the body is stretched and hangs completely from the straight arms with the head bent backward (Cobra).
7. On exhalation, move the body back again in the same way till it rests in the Hare, with the forehead and the arms on the floor.
8. During inhalation raise first the arms, keeping them straight, then the head, and then the whole upper part of the body to sitting position. The order is important as it forces you to use the muscles in the small of the back.
9. Lower the arms, keeping them straight,

10. The Best pose
Lie on the stomach with the legs a little apart.

Lie with the head turned to one side. The elbows are pointing out to the sides and the hands are clasped over the ear. Lie five minutes or more. After some time, turn the head to the other side.

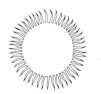

Hatha Yoga

For theory on the **cleansing techniques** see the section on *Hatha Yoga* in Chapter 5, which is about the different branches of the tradition.

1. Neti, Nose Cleansing

Neti is a Hatha Yoga cleansing process. By cleansing the mucous membranes in the nose, they are stimulated so that the surrounding area is strengthened - including the eyebrow centre which is an important point of contact

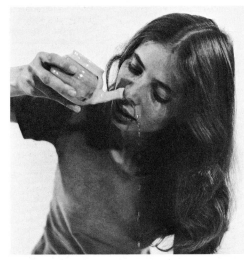

for the *Ajna Chakra*, the third eye, or, physiologically, the pineal gland. The entire breathing system is affected by Neti. The little cilia hairs which clean the air passages by "sweeping" up the dirt are also activated as the mucous membranes are affected. So we have the best conceivable exercise against the effects of air pollution. This is reinforced by the breathing exercise that follows Neti,

Blacksmith's Bellows (*Bhastrika*), which also cleans and oxygenates the blood, thereby bringing greater clarity to the brain.

Neti

Take a little cup with a spout (perhaps a teapot), fill it with warm water (approx. 1/2 pint, not too warm) and dissolve one teaspoon of salt in it. Lean forward and tilt your head to one side. Place the spout in the upper nostril, keep your mouth open and breathe in a relaxed way through your mouth. Pour the water into your nose very carefully, so that it runs out through the other nostril. Your head should not be tilted too far to the side, just held at an angle, so that the water will run out easily. Repeat the whole process leaning to the other side.

When you have finished, close one nostril with a finger and blow out gently through the other several times, doing both sides until the nose is dry and clean. Note: Never close both nostrils simultaneously when you blow the nose. Stand for a while with your head hanging down or do the Clown (page 46), so the water can run out of the nose. Afterwards do the Blacksmith's Bellows (page 49).

2. Kapalabhati, the Bellows that cleans the frontal part of the brain

Sit in a meditation pose and close your eyes.

1. Breathe out short and fast, and let air be inhaled automatically. Exhale by pulling in your stomach muscles. Imagine that the air is shooting up through the top of your head.
   When you inhale, you don't have to think about the breath, just let the air flow in by itself. Exhale each time with a sudden, short and powerful movement. Relax fully while inhaling, so that you get enough air. Do between thirty and a hundred fast exhalations, then:

2. Exhale completely - empty yourself of air, bend your neck so that your chin touches your chest, keep your breath out, pull up your sex-organs, perineum and anus and suck up your

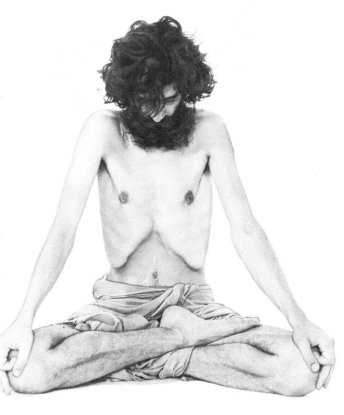

stomach (Chin Lock, Root Lock and Abdominal Lock, page 82). Hold your breath out as long as you can while concentrating - up through the top of your head - on emptiness. Before you inhale, first relax all contractions and raise the head. Normally repeated three times.
   If you become too hot during this exercise, do it in a more relaxed way - and perhaps use one of the cooling breathing methods afterwards (page 80).
   Kapalabhati cleans the air passages, the bronchial passages and nose. It gets rid of depressions and tensions in the brain.

3. Tratak

Intense concentration. See chapter 10: Inspired Interest.

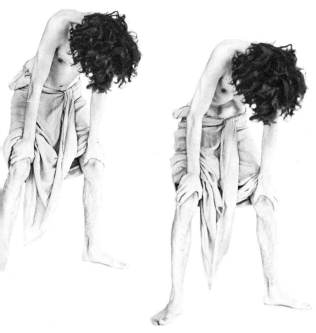

4. That which Kindles the Fire

The digestive fire.

This exercise must be learned in four steps:

1. Stand with your legs apart. Lean forward, resting your hands on your slightly bent knees, look down at your stomach and move it in and out gently, and without straining, twenty times.

2. Do this while breathing in and out twenty times.

3. Exhale completely, steady your hands on your knees, bend your neck so that your chin touches your chest, hold your breath out, using the vacuum to suck up your stomach so it forms a cavity under your ribs. Hold this as long as you can. Your ribs will protrude sharply and your stomach will be drawn up and back at an angle, not straight back, with a relaxed abdomen. Master this before going on.

4. Kindling the Fire

After you have sucked up your stomach, go on holding your breath out. Then relax your stomach, let it drop and then pull it up again, up and down, lightly and easily, as many times as you can.

Finally relax your lower abdomen again, relax your throat, straighten up and breathe in.

The Kindling of the Fire improves digestion and strengthens the digestive organs; it also provides relief from stress.

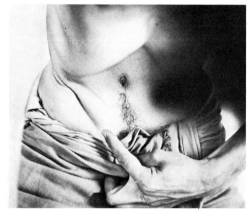

5. Nauli

Rotation of the abdominal muscles.

1. Like 3 in exercise **4**. Hold your breath out and suck up your stomach while you support your hands on your knees.

2. Get a little tendon to appear out on one side of the abdominal cavity. The tendon will stand out when you place your weight on the hand (and knee) on the same side. Do it on the other side too. Note: You may not achieve this all at once, but master it before you proceed with the following steps.

3. Now move this little tendon futher towards the center of the cavity by putting more weight on the hand and relaxing the surrounding area where the muscle comes forward. It will then appear as a slightly thicker muscle on that side of the abdomen. This is done while you hold your breath out. Do the same on the other side.

4. Now produce a thicker muscle in the centre of the abdomen by pressing both hands equally on both knees.

5. Let the pressure shift from one knee to the other - and get the muscle to "rotate": forward in the centre, to one side, back (hollowing), to the other side, the centre again, to the side, etc.

This is *Nauli*, which awakens the psychic energy at the navel area and keeps the abdomen free from disease, tensions and stress.

When you start learning this and the preceding exercises, do them in the morning before breakfast - but after you have been to the toilet - and eat as little as you can as early as possible the evening before.

After That which Kindles the Fire and Nauli you should always rest on your back for **at least three minutes.**

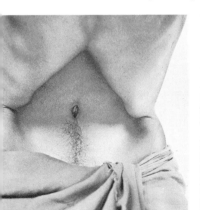
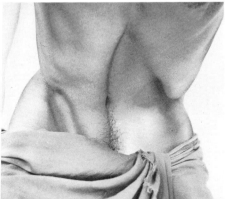
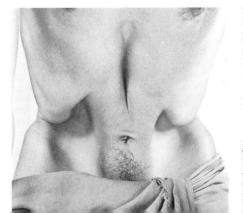
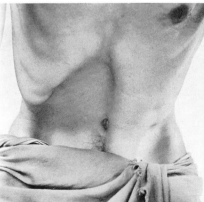

Loosening the Knots / Shakti Bandha

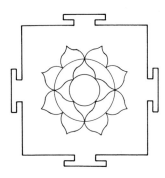

who moves through the Sushumna channel in the spinal cord to reach Shiva, fully-awakened consciousness, her masculine opposite pole, residing in the *Sahasrara Chakra* in the upper part of the head.

The union of and harmony between these polarities, the masculine and feminine, is called yoga. This programme releases tensions that hinder the energy from flowing freely.

She is the light itself and transcendent.
From her body proceed thousand,
two thousand, hundred thousand, ten million,
hundreds of millions of beams - it is
not possible to know their great number.
It is she who causes all things
to radiate, those that stand still
and those that move.
By this goddess' light
all things appear.

(Bhairava-Yamala)

Most of the postures in this programme are done in the Diamond pose (*Vajrasana*). They are sitting-still poses designed for absorption, concentration and relaxation. You will get the best experience and the greatest profit if you do the whole programme without a break. Remain in the Diamond pose all the time, and go from one exercise straight into the next. It may be hard for beginners to do the programme this way - if so, rest between the different exercises and stretch your legs. Still, in order to keep the intensity, it is important not to lie down and relax until the whole programme is finished.

Shakti

Shakti is the body's energy or power. *Bandha* means to contract (bind, lock) or tighten, in this case a knot (block). Shakti is also the power found in the root chakra, the energy centre above the perineum, Muladhara Chakra. Here it is said that the *Kundalini Shakti*, in the form of a snake, lies coiled three and a half times around an oval shaped form (page 15 and chapter 8).

In Tantra this energy is described symbolically as Shakti, the primal female energy, the "primal mother", the goddess

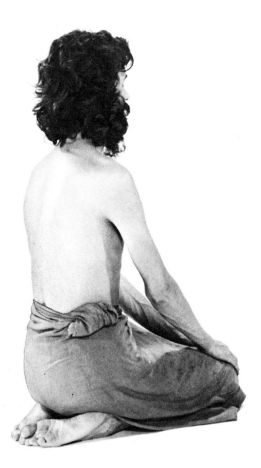

The Diamond pose

Sit back on your lower legs, knees together, so that your big toes touch and your heels turn out to the side, your feet forming a "bowl" for your buttocks to rest in. Place your hands on your knees. Keep your spine (and the small of your back) straight and your head upright. This pose has various effects:

1. Physically it has a beneficial effect on the liver and digestion. So it is good to sit in the pose after meals for ten to fifteen minutes. The Diamond pose is the one posture that can be assumed without discomfort immediately after eating - with the other poses you should wait three to four hours.

This pose is also good for the pelvis and the entire spine, as the spine is held straight at the small of the back, where most people commonly slump when they sit any length of time. Muscle pain in the knees, calves and thighs is diminished by regular use of this pose. Relieves sciatica.

2. For meditation the Diamond pose is very good, even though at first the legs are apt to fall asleep. This is not "dangerous", just slightly uncomfortable. However, when you have been sitting in the pose for some time, come out of it slowly and carefully.

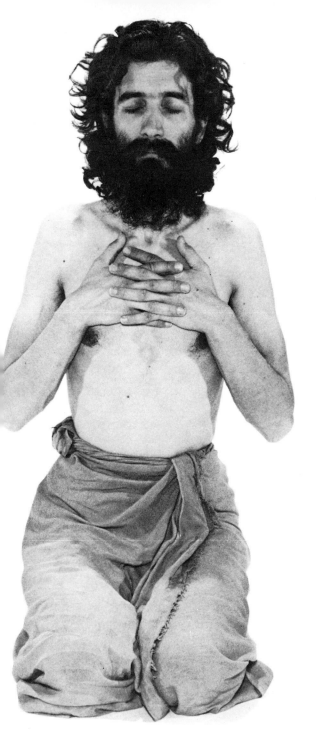

1. Tuning in to Going Deeper

Sit in the Diamond pose with your hands clasped on your chest and your eyes closed. Experience the body:

1. Feel the crown of the head - forehead - eyes - nose - cheeks - jaws - mouth. Feel the top part of the back of your head - nape of your neck - throat - your whole head.
Experience your arms - upper arms - elbows - lower arms. Chest - back - whole back - whole upper torso. Experience or feel your stomach - small of the back - abdomen - buttocks. Thighs - knees - lower legs. Ankles - heels - soles - ball of the foot - instep - both soles.

2. Experience the body as a whole.

3. For a long while experience just your hands.

4. The whole body.

5. The whole body and its natural breathing.

Relaxing. Increases sensitivity and your ability to experience your body. 5-10 minutes. Could be extended indefinitely.

2. Attention on the Tip of your Nose

Sit in the Diamond pose with your hands on your knees.

A. Start with eyes closed.
1. Think of the tip of your nose.
2. Sense it.
3. Feel it from within. Sit this way for a while with eyes closed, keeping your attention on the tip of your nose.

B. Open your eyes, gaze at your nose tip, squint, focus all your attention on your nose, try to see the tip clearly and equally with both eyes. When your eyes tire or your attention wanders return to **A**, close your eyes. When your attention wanders with your eyes closed or you feel the need to open them, open your eyes again and look at the nose tip (**B**). Alternate between **A** and **B** for 5-10 minutes or longer.

Gazing at your nose tip is called *Nasikagra Drishti* in Sanskrit and is part of many advanced exercises.

Concentrating. Used in Kundalini Yoga in connection with Ajna chakra behind the eyebrow centre, and Muladhara chakra. If breathing through your nose is difficult, sit with your arms crossed over your chest, tuck your hands up into the armpits, and press your hands with the upper arms, thumbs pointing up in front of your shoulders and the rest of the hand under your arms. This will open your nostrils.

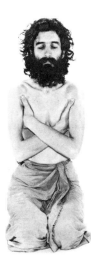

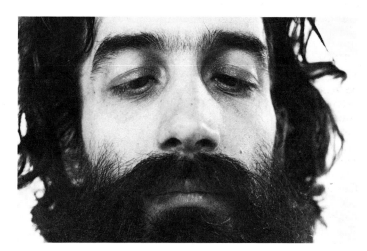

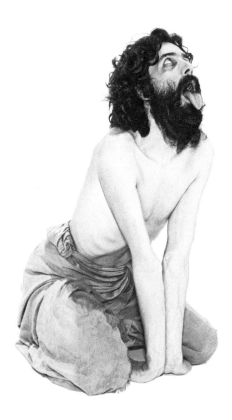

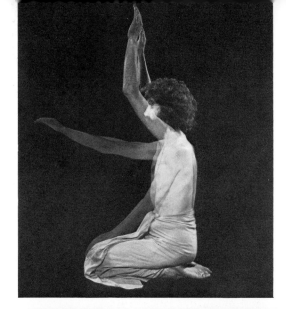

Relaxing. The Lion has a strengthening effect on the voice. Some speech teachers use it to cure stuttering. It counteracts diseases of the ears, nose, eyes and throat. Tensions in these areas are released.

By keeping your attention fixed on the eyebrow centre, you create a calming and concentrating effect. This is a very powerful preparation for meditation.

4. Breathing and Movements Go Together

Sit in the Diamond pose with your hands on your knees.

1. Inhale while raising your arms straight over your head. The movement and breath should be simultaneous and as slow as possible.

2. Bend your upper body forward until your arms and head touch the floor, as you exhale. Exhalation should start with the movement, follow it, ending when the movement is completed.

3. Hold your breath as long as you can.

4. Then raise your arms and body while inhaling. Breathe and move as slowly as possible.

5. Exhale and place your hands on your knees.

Pause and come to rest before repeating the exercise. The whole cycle should be repeated seven times with pauses between. It is important for the breathing and movements to be done together and for it all to be as slow as possible.

Concentrating. In this exercise you learn to control your breathing and movements. As you come to master it, it will have a very calming effect and steady the nervous system, make you aware of restlessness and counteract it.

Breathing and Movement go Together prepares you for more advanced breathing exercises.

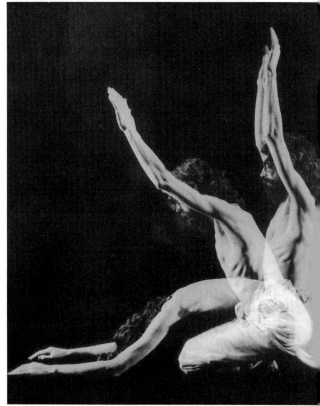

3. The Lion's Roar

Sit in the Diamond pose with your legs apart. Place your palms on the floor between your knees, fingers pointing in towards your body, thumbs out to each side. Part of your weight now rests on your arms. Become slightly swayback. Look up towards the eyebrow centre. Inhale, then bend your head as far back as you can. Stick your tongue far out towards your chin and make the kind of sound you do for a doctor, "aaah...", but much louder, deeper, and for as long as possible. It is important to look at the eyebrow centre while the tongue is out.

Relax after each "roar" in the Diamond pose, with closed eyes. Remember to wait to bend your head back until you have inhaled.

"Roar" this way seven times.

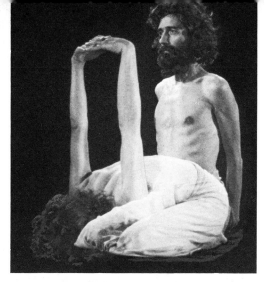

3. Bend forward until your forehead touches the floor and:

4. Raise your arms until your clasped hands are right over your shoulders. Arms, hands and shoulders form a firm frame which:

5. Is swung from side to side, as long as you can hold your breath. If you do this correctly, one of your shoulders will touch one of your knees, or be in front of it, every time "the frame" swings to one side.

6. Then straighten up to a sitting position, lower your arms and exhale.

7. Pause, let your whole organism come to rest, experience this sitting with your eyes closed. Then inhale and repeat the exercise.

This may be hard to do and could require instruction from a teacher. The swings can be fast or slow, depending on how powerful an effect you want. For some people, it helps to separate the knees slightly.

Relaxing. Shakti Bandha dissolves tensions in the spine and thereby enables psychic energy to flow freely.

5. Loosening the Knots "Shakti Bandha"

1. Sit in the Diamond pose. Clasp your hands behind your back.

2. Inhale.

6. The Camel

This is done in three variations:

A. 1. Kneel with your hands on your waist, thumbs forward, fingers pointing back.

2. Take a deep breath and then exhale while you lean your head and the upper part of your body back, pushing your hips forward. While you stay in this pose, breathe gently. Hold the pose a while (one half to two minutes) and focus on Manipura Chakra, from your navel area and backward to the spine.

3. Then straighten up again.

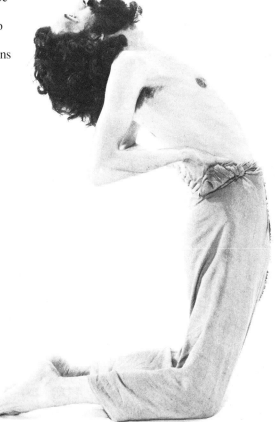

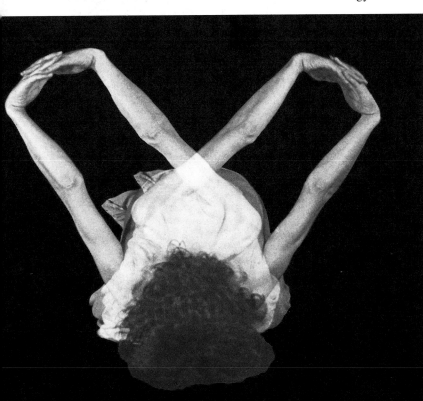

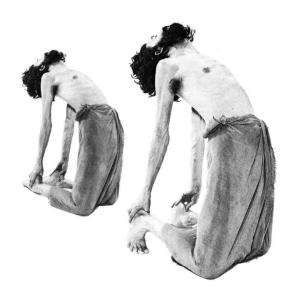

8. The Bumble Bee

The breathing exercise associated with Shakti Bandha is called the Bumble Bee. Sit in a meditation pose. Inhale deeply through both nostrils, hold your breath and bend your head so your chin rests on your chest in the Chin Lock. Contract the anus, perenium and sex organs - the Root Lock - while relaxing the rest of your body and face. (See also page 82.)

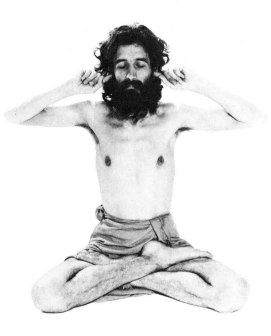

B. Do this exercise as in **A** but instead of keeping your hands at your waist, rest them on your heels, your feet vertical with your toes on the floor.

C. As **B** but keep feet and ankles on the floor.

The Camel strengthens the lower abdomen and intestines, it is good for stooping backs and relieves back pains.

7. Dead Still

Lie stretched out on your back with legs slightly parted and arms and hands comfortably by your sides. Lie still for at least five to ten minutes. Direct your attention to the body, its contour and form. After a while experience natural breathing, especially in your nose. All the time be aware that you are lying perfectly still. **Relaxing.**

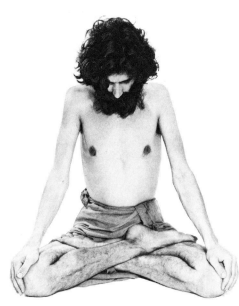

Let your hands rest on your knees and your body weight rest lightly on your arms. Hold your breath briefly in this position.

Then relax the Root Lock, raise your head, relax your shoulders and exhale.

When you exhale, it is done through your nose. Your mouth is closed with parted teeth. Close your ears with a finger in each, holding your arms at shoulder level. Now exhale with a low powerful hum. Your eyes remain closed. Feel that you become one with the sound vibration, let the sound fill you, your head and more. And experience: "This is my sound, this is me, I can form myself by forming this sound."

Do the Bumble Bee seven times or as many times you like.

Relaxing and Concentrating. The Bumble Bee is a breathing exercise that dissolves tensions in the brain caused by anger. It lowers high blood pressure caused by mental irritation and is a valuable discipline for musicians. Used as a warm-up for Nada Yoga (pages 68 and 83).

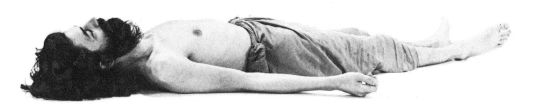

Eye Yoga

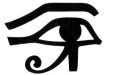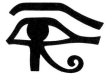

The sight is controlled by muscles. **Muscles** move the eye so it can see in different directions. Muscles are tightened and relaxed and so influence the form of the eye. We can finely tune the sight to read a book, to talk to another human being or to watch when we move about in traffic.

Near-sightedness can be due to a permanent tension in those muscles that make the eye longer and thinner. Normally we use these muscles to focus on things nearby.

Far-sightedness can be due to a permanent tension in those muscles that make the form of the eye short and thick and help us to see things far away.

The yoga eye exercises influence the sight by making the musculature of the eyes more supple. This is as simple as it sounds: **Train your eyesight and see better!**

Naturally our **state** influences how well we see. When we are stressed, tired or worried, our sight is not as good as it is under normal conditions. Some find that their vision worsens when they have had a cup of coffee, while they see much better after a relaxation or after yoga exercises. The energy level of the eyes has an effect too. Through different exercises the eyes can become used to more energy, being more concentrated and more relaxed.

Our **attitude** towards what we are looking at is also important. Have you ever tried to read a book with fully relaxed eyes? It is quite obvious that you cannot keep as critical a distance from what you are reading as you usually do. A critical attitude is often

reflected in the expression on the face. We squint our eyes and raise the head a bit. Is it a defensive attitude, a wish not to be invaded by an opinion, by an influence from another human being, or by something we experience?

In other words, by using certain exercises and by realizing our own attitude to the world around us, we can learn to influence our sight. In the open state that we experience during a relaxation or meditation, the mind will not react and we can effectively use a visualization or a resolution like: "My sight is getting better and better", and thus create a new possibility in our subconscious.

A very important eye exercise is *Tratak*, which we will go through in chapter 10. It is worth using along with the other exercises. If you want to do all the exercises that improve your sight this is a good sequence: nose cleansing (see the text on Hatha Yoga page 56), yoga poses (especially Head Rolling page 36, Standing Swinging pose page 47, the Clown page 46, and Headstand page 70 - choose one at a time), the eye exercises used in this chapter, Tratak and finally the Yoga Nidra relaxation, either that on page 98, or another, deeper version on my guided cassette tape *Experience Yoga Nidra*.

Even though we may see better right after a relaxation - test it yourself - we may lose some of it again when we are subjected to daily stress. Therefore it pays to repeat the yoga eye exercises suggested here - and your sight will gradually improve.

Eye exercises

If you use glasses or contact lenses, you should remove them when you do the exercises explained below. Whenever you can do without your glasses, even if you don't see clearly in the beginning, take them off and give your eyes a chance to see for themselves.

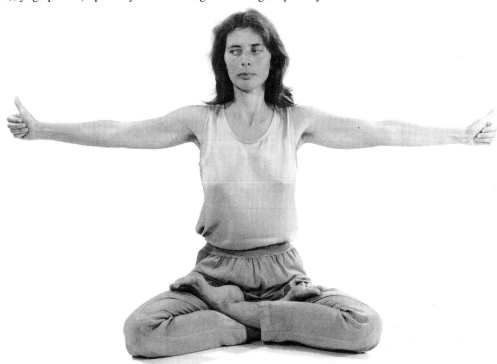

Move the eyes in all directions

Place yourself comfortably on a chair or on the floor. Take time to do the exercises, and do them all in a relaxed way.

1. Stretch your arms out to the sides with the thumbs pointing upward. Keep your head still and your face turned forward. Look alternately from one thumb to the other, only by turning the eyes towards the thumbs. Do the movement about 15 times. Gradually you may be able to turn the eyes more and more to the sides without straining, and thus expand your field of vision. Therefore, keep the arms out straight and as far back as you can so that you can only see the thumbs at the edge of your field of vision. Then close the eyes and sit still for a minute or so and relax.

2. Keep the head still. Stretch one arm upward until the thumb is at the edge of your field of vision, and the other arm downward to the lower edge of your vision. Look from one thumb to the other, up and down about 15 times. Then close the eyes and relax.

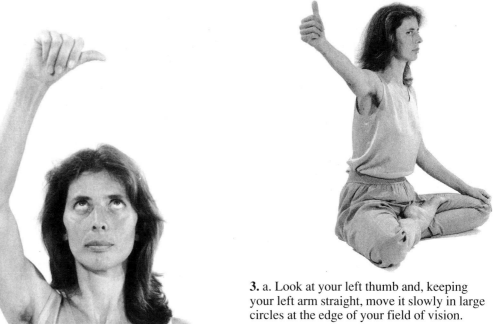

3. a. Look at your left thumb and, keeping your left arm straight, move it slowly in large circles at the edge of your field of vision. Don't move your head as you do this. Move your arm one way around 5 times and then the other way around 5 times. Do this with the right thumb as well.

   b. Draw the number eight as big as possible several times, vertical and horizontal. Keep the head still, so that only the eyes follow the movement of the thumb.

   c. Draw squares with their corners extending all the way to the border of your field of vision. The arm is straight all the time.

   d. Draw all kinds of pointed edged figures with your thumb: five-pointed stars, triangles pointing upward, inverted triangles... Keep reaching the edge of your field of vision.

All the muscles that move the eyes have now been moved and trained and the optic nerves have been stimulated. Before we go to the focal exercises, we must rest the eyes:

Rest and nourish the eyes

4. Rub your palms with small quick movements against each other until they become quite warm. Then place the warm palms across the cavities of the eyes with the fingers placed on top of each other on the forehead. Make sure that you can open and close the eyes under the palms without any problems and with no light coming through. Sit for a moment and feel the heat flow from your hands into your eyes while you rest them. Imagine that your eyes are soft and receptive. You can support your elbows on your knees if you sit on the floor, or if you sit on a chair you can place them on a table.

Focus

5. Keep one arm straight out in front of you, with the thumb pointing upward. Look at the thumb while you move it in towards the point between the eyebrows and back again. Move the thumb back and forth 10-20 times at a slow and steady speed. If you are near-sighted or far-sighted, you may not be able to see the thumb clearly all the way, but do the whole movement anyway, straightening your arm fully and bringing your thumb right back to the eyebrow centre.

6. Keep one arm straight out in front of you with the thumb pointing upward, and bend the other with the thumb placed in the middle between the first thumb and the tip of your nose. Alternatively look at the tip of your nose, the nearest thumb, the farthest thumb and a point further away. Focus as clearly as possible on each of these points 10-20 times.

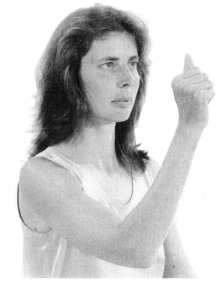

Now rest the eyes again, as described under point **4.**

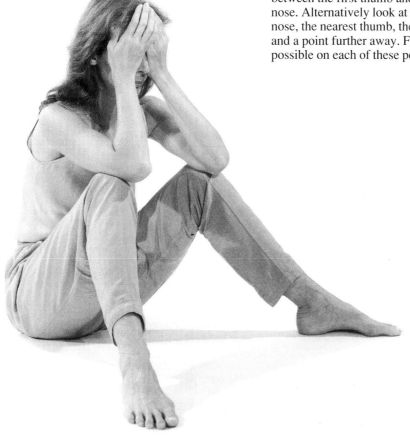

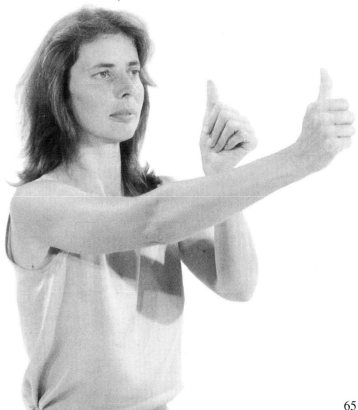

65

Reach deeper

7. When in a calm manner you hold a muscle stretched for a while, the tension in the muscle will be reduced and the energy previously bound there will be released. This happens in the yoga poses, and it happens when without turning the head, you let your eyes look at a point for some time at the edge of your field of vision. Keep looking at a point to the side, up or down. Roll the eyes (exercise 8) to find those points or angles where there is languidness or where it hurts a little, then keep the eyes in that position.

8. Roll the eyes 10 times, first one way and then the other. Don't think about how to move the eyes, instead look around along the edge of your field of vision - in a continuous movement, without stopping anywhere. This exercise is important also in advanced yoga, as it releases fundamental tensions, and thus strengthens the total state of your energy. Do it in a calm manner and only after you have warmed up with exercises **1 - 6.**

9. Squint and look at the eyebrow center, hold the gaze there for a moment, then squint and look at the tip of your nose for a moment. Move back and forth several times between the two points. This exercise removes deeper seated tensions, not only in the eyes, but in the whole body. Don't overdo it, do it only after the previous exercises and before the next. With a bit of practice you can hold your gaze fixed longer and longer at the two points.

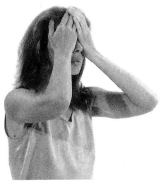

Rest and Relax

Now rest for about 10 minutes with the exercise described under point **4**. Rub your hands time and again during this sitting. Or:

Sit with closed eyes and your face turned towards the morning sun. Let the sun shine on your eyelids for about five minutes. Then place your hand over the eyes for about five minutes as described in **4.**

Take some time to lie on your back and look up at the sky at a time of the day when the light is not too strong. Stay there until you feel quite calm and feel your eyes are soft without focusing on anything. Or look over a landscape for a long while.

If you want to do more than this then carry on with **Tratak**, which has a strong cleansing, concentrating and energizing effect (page 103).

When you look at something, you don't need to strain to get the sight impression into your eyes. Do not look **with** the eyes, look **through** the eyes. They are your windows; the sight impression will come by itself.

The Ladder

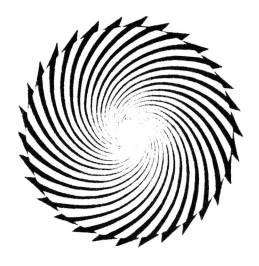

Attitudes

With this course of exercises, we come to an area of yoga different from and complementary to both the breathing exercises and the poses. These are called attitudes.

An attitude, in Sanskrit called *mudra,* is an exercise which produces a deep inward effect. It influences the underlying form or state of energy in and around your body. An apparently slight physical influence unblocks the subtle energy currents and makes them flow harmoniously. This relaxes different areas of the body. Thus the attitudes or postures influence the nervous system and the chakras, energizing or awakening the corresponding areas in the brain.

This book contains two programmes of attitudes, the Ladder on the following pages, and the Deep Ones starting on page 82.

Most of the exercises in the Ladder can relieve different forms of headaches.

Start by sitting still with eyes closed.

1. The Mare

Variation 1:
Slowly tighten your anus, hold it drawn in and up for a while and then slowly relax it completely. Do this twenty-five times or more. Do it as slowly as possible.

Variation 2:
1. Slowly draw your anus in and up while you inhale.
2. Hold these muscles and your breath as long as you can.
3. Slowly relax as you exhale; relax completely. Inhale, repeating the process.

Afterwards remain sitting relaxed for a while with closed eyes, and concentrate on *Muladhara Chakra*, just above the perineum.

Then proceed to exercise 2.

The Mare increases the blood supply, cures constipation, prevents haemorrhoids and loss of energy due to hypotension.

2. Thunderbolt

The thunderbolt is the name of a psychic current in the body that supplies the sexual organs with sensitivity and energy.

Pull up your sexual organs by tensing them and contracting the urinary tract - like holding back urine before urinating. The testicles or vagina should be included in this, it may feel like the contraction is centered just above the sexual organs. Do it slowly without straining - drawing upward while you inhale. Don't pull the anus at the same time (difficult, but try anyway). Hold it as long as you can hold your breath and then slowly relax as you exhale.

Concentrate on *Swadhisthana Chakra*, start at the contact area around the sex organs and move to the chakra itself, at the base of the spine.

The Thunderbolt releases tensions in the sexual organs and gives greater vitality and control to the area. If you want to refrain from sex, this exercise helps. It is an important pre-paration for the Tantric sexual ritual, and is good for a normal sex life: you avoid tensions during intercourse and convert energy that might otherwise become blocked (Chapter 7).

3. The Water Jug

1. Extend your legs in front of you and grasp your big toes.
2. Inhale, pushing your stomach out as far as you can - hold your breath and your stomach out as long as you can. Keep your back as straight as possible without straining.
3. Exhale and relax a moment with closed eyes, then repeat the exercise - up to nine times. If you need to, let go of the toes between rounds.

Concentrate on *Manipura Chakra* behind your navel.

The Water Jug is an important exercise to strengthen the bowels. It relaxes the whole navel-stomach area and reduces stress. It also makes you clear headed.

Don't do it right after going to the toilet.

4. The Space of the Heart

Sit relaxed in a meditation pose with closed eyes (see page 84 and 85).

Experience your natural breathing, how your inhalation flows from your nose or throat to an empty space that you discover in your heart area. This space is called *space of the heart*. It has no distinct limits but has its starting points around the heart. Feel how every inhalation expands this space. Go deeply into the concentration without straining - it's no good if you strain - and keep sensing how your breath fills this space.

Note: This is not a physical expansion of the chest - just breathe normally and relax. This exercise is directly related to *Anahata Chakra*, behind the heart; it creates relaxation in the heart and breathing.

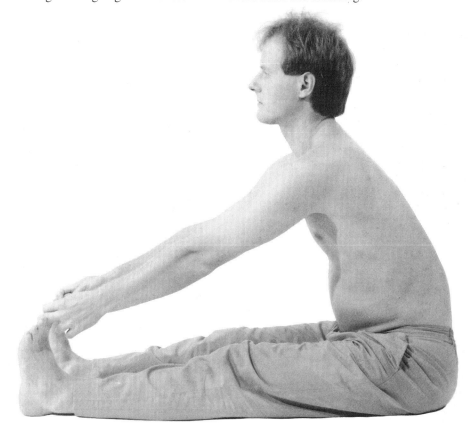

5. Psychic Breathing

This is done with your tongue curled up and back and your attention focused on *Vishuddhi Chakra* at the throat (page 49).

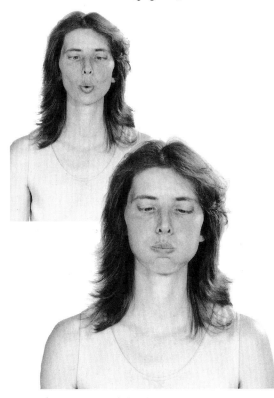

6. The Crow

1. Purse your lips and let the breath slowly stream in through this hole with a slight sound. Notice a cool feeling in your mouth. Gaze at the tip of your nose.
2. Hold your breath and puff out your cheeks for a while. Keep looking at the tip of your nose.
3. Close your eyes, relax your cheeks and exhale through your nostrils.
4. Inhale again with open eyes. Do this sequence up to nine times or more.

This relaxes your head psychically, eliminates mouth and throat diseases and improves digestion by increasing glandular secretion.

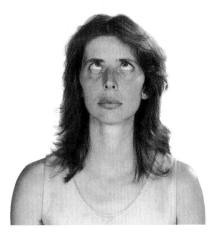

7. Gazing at the Eyebrow Centre

Look up cross-eyed at the centre between your eyebrows (3-5 minutes). Rest your eyes occasionally.

This relaxes the nerves and affects *Ajna Chakra* behind the eyebrow centre.

8. The Sound

Straddle a mat or a cushion, close your ears with your thumbs, close your eyes and listen inwardly to *Bindu*, the point at the top of the back of your head. You'll hear different sounds, one after another; keep listening for the subtlest and newest and, when that is clear, proceed to the next more subtle and indistinct one. Go on as long as you like.

Sounds can be like: whistling, murmuring, flutes, high frequency transmissions, clocks, music, surf, crickets, songs.

This exercise is a brief introduction to the very important form of meditation called *Nada Yoga* - sound yoga. It results in great psychic and mental relaxation and is practised at night when it is dark, if the sound cannot be heard in the day.

If you have been hearing high frequency sounds before you got to know yoga and didn't know what to make of it, you may benefit from transforming the sounds through this exercise (also see page 22). However, if you resist hearing these sounds, don't do the exercise.

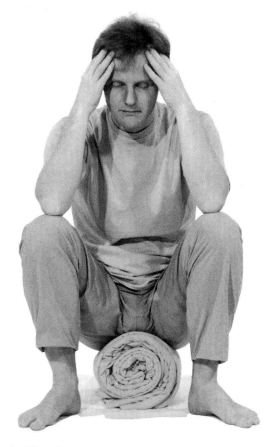

9. The Space

Experience a space in your head, an empty space that you fill with your consciousness, your awareness. You are this space, experience it - its walls, ceiling, floor, etc. - feel it from within. Keep at it for a while and then go on to the next exercise.

10. The Flame

Experience a fire, a flaming fire, burning from the top of your head. Experience it as a great flame burning up from your crown. Then sit still for a while before opening your eyes and looking round.

The Classical Programme

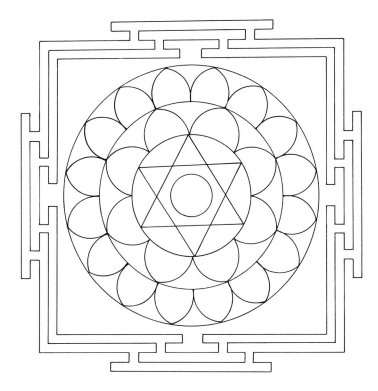

This programme consists of some of the best known, most profoundly effective poses. The **sequence** of this programme is very exactly determined. The order in which the poses are practised is not accidental. They are presented in two variations: a long course, which has a stronger effect, and a short one which I recommend you use to start your training.

The pictures and text show the long programme and the sequence of the short course is described afterwards (page 79).

The poses are also linked together in subgroups, **poses** and **counterposes**, e.g. Headstand (on your head) and the Palm (on your feet) or the Back Stretch (bending forward) and the Abdominal Stretch (bending backward). If you want the best possible effect, these combinations must be adhered to.

The programme may be carried out in several ways:

1. The learning phase. Follow the instructions carefully and train your body to be able to sit or stand in the poses.

2. When you have mastered the individual poses quite well (you really don't have to be a perfectionist: go as far as you can and be patient - they'll still be effective), and when you can relax in the poses, then **put the programme together** so that you begin to experience it as an ongoing sequence.

3. Move slowly and steadily into a pose and **experience the way you move your body.** Every movement should be done and felt consciously. Hold the pose. Then come slowly and precisely out of the pose again.

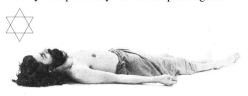

4. Pause between poses. Between two counterposes there is seldom a break, but between the different groups of poses, pause on your back.

Experience this pause as mindfully as possible: experience your body coming to rest - breathing, pulse, nerves, the whole body. Become aware of a "zero point" at the moment of attaining complete calm - and, just before you start getting restless or your mind wanders or you get sleepy, then go on to the next pose.

5. Experience motionlessness in a pose. What is it like to stay absolutely still? Gather your whole attention around motionlessness and stay still in each pose as long as instructed, without moving in the least, and experience it - relaxed motionlessness.

6. Experience movements. The different poses and the whole programme can be done with many varied movements as a dynamic programme by going into and out of a pose several times, e.g. by swinging your legs, thus paying greater attention to the physical effect - this can be physically refreshing.

7. Experience the chakras. In both the long and the short programmes we are concerned with poses which, besides the many physical effects, also have psychic effects such as the ability to achieve peacefulness, balance and greater depth. This is enhanced when you focus your attention on a single point or a smaller area during each pose. Like the steps in "Sun, I greet you", each pose has, as its point of concentration, a chakra located in the spinal cord. Concentrate on the corresponding chakra when you are in a pose. The whole subject of chakras is so important that we will discuss it in a separate chapter. First learn the poses. Then read chapter 8 on the different chakras.

Warm up with the "Sun, I greet you" (page 28) or the Triangle poses (page 44). Then start right off with the first pose given here:

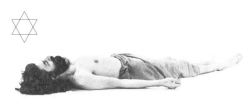

1. Dead Still

A relaxation pose
used after "Sun, I greet you"
and as a preparation for this programme.

The mind comes to rest,
the body comes to rest,
the whole person becomes attuned to
doing the exercises.
This is one of the most important yogic poses.
Lie on your back
with your arms by your sides,
your legs straight next to each other,
slightly apart.
Sink into a completely calm state,
lie for a while experiencing your whole body,
the whole form of your body.
In this way, prepare for the programme.

When you have done the following poses enough times and you know them well enough that you can picture yourself doing them correctly, then **lie with your eyes closed and see yourself in the poses**. This can be a great help in the way you progress with yoga.

Dead Still is a very important yoga pose. Do it every time it is mentioned in the course of this programme.
   Then proceed to the next exercise.

2. The Headstand

This pose cannot be over-valued. No person who practises yoga will know the true effect of yoga until he/she has mastered the Headstand.
   To prepare for it, use the Clown, page 47.

1. Kneel and place your forearms on the floor with your hands at a distance in front of your knees, your fingers interlocked. Your elbows should be far enough apart for your forearms to form the sides of an equilateral triangle. If your elbows are too far apart, you can fall backwards and if they are too close, you may fall to one side.

2. Place your head in your hands with your crown resting on the mat; place it firmly, so that it will not roll.

3. Straighten your legs and go forward on your toes until the upper part of your body is vertical.

4. Inhale, hold your breath, bend your legs, lifting your feet off the floor. Balance yourself before you go further, with the weight of your body now completely divided between your head and arms.

5. Lift your feet so that they rise over your buttocks.

6. Slowly extend your legs upwards. Now the body is standing straight and vertical. Breathe normally.

Note: If you should fall backwards, roll quickly into a ball by bending your neck as you would in a somersault. Thus you will avoid thudding onto the floor with your feet and hitting your back. Always do this pose where you won't fall onto something or hit yourself - at first you might try it against a wall, but become independent of the wall soon as it may result in an incorrect pose.

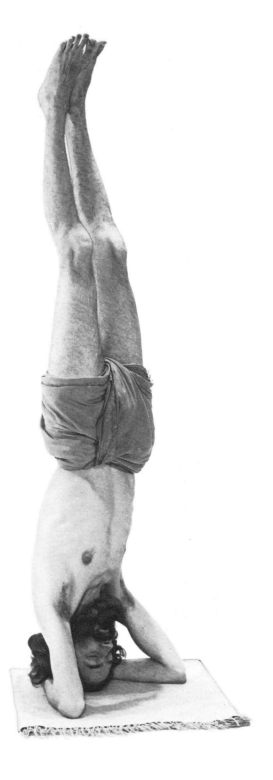

Concentrate on Sahasrara Chakra at the top of your head - it covers the crown, the brain and the hair above. Relax your body without letting the pose become slack - especially relax the abdomen.

This pose should not be done by people with high blood pressure without expert guidance, or by those who have suffered a cerebral haemorrhage or have a weak heart. It is good for the brain, the heart and the circulatory system, for psychic balance and reducing anxiety; for the legs and glands, for the sexual organs; against headaches, asthma, hay fever, lethargy, depression. The whole body is helped by the Headstand, the most important of all yoga poses.

Eventually you can stay in the Headstand as long as you like (half an hour). The norm is five minutes but start with one minute.

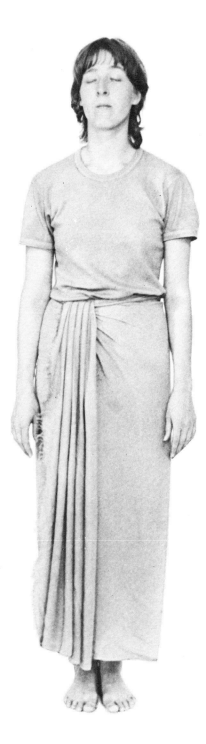

2. Make different leg movements like parting your legs sideways or back and forwards. Also arch your body by pushing out your stomach and pulling your feet back.
3. When you have completely mastered the Headstand, bring your legs into the Lotus pose.

3. The Palm

Counterpose to the Headstand.

Stand with your arms raised up over your head, hands clasped, palms up. Inhale, go up on your toes, look up at your hands and balance for a while. Then come down again on to your soles, lower your arms, exhale and stand for a moment relaxed. However, if you do the Headstand for a long time (three minutes or more), do the Palm in a relaxed way, standing normally with closed eyes and your arms at your sides.

For constipation, drink some lukewarm water and walk around on your toes in this pose a while.

Concentration: Sahasrara Chakra at the top of the head. See also the Palm, page 47.

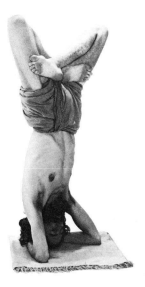

Variations:
1. Go from the Clown directly up into the Headstand keeping the same arm position.

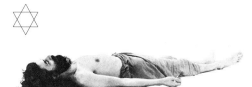

Pause in Dead Still for one and a half to two minutes.

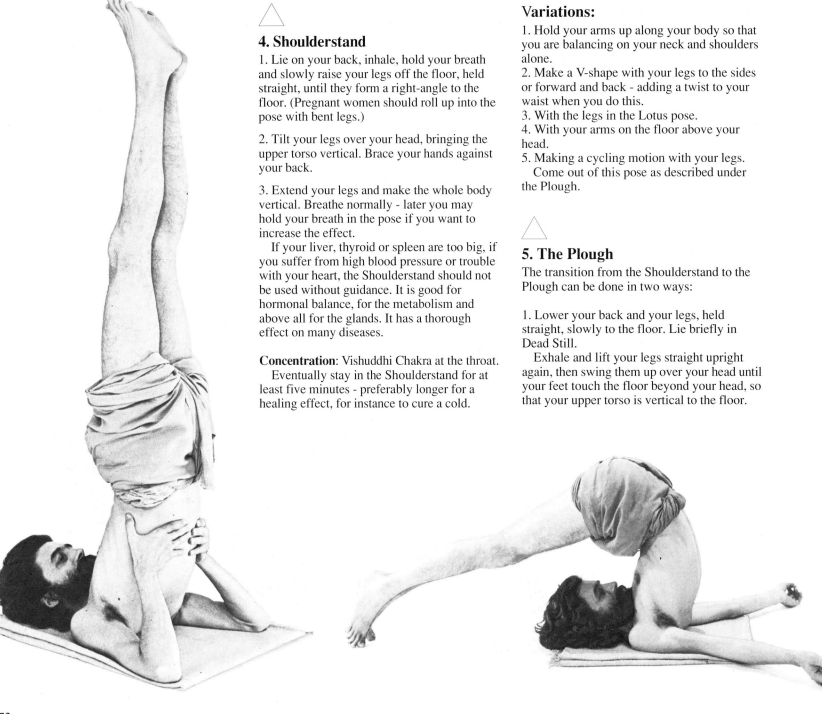

4. Shoulderstand

1. Lie on your back, inhale, hold your breath and slowly raise your legs off the floor, held straight, until they form a right-angle to the floor. (Pregnant women should roll up into the pose with bent legs.)

2. Tilt your legs over your head, bringing the upper torso vertical. Brace your hands against your back.

3. Extend your legs and make the whole body vertical. Breathe normally - later you may hold your breath in the pose if you want to increase the effect.
    If your liver, thyroid or spleen are too big, if you suffer from high blood pressure or trouble with your heart, the Shoulderstand should not be used without guidance. It is good for hormonal balance, for the metabolism and above all for the glands. It has a thorough effect on many diseases.

Concentration: Vishuddhi Chakra at the throat.
    Eventually stay in the Shoulderstand for at least five minutes - preferably longer for a healing effect, for instance to cure a cold.

Variations:

1. Hold your arms up along your body so that you are balancing on your neck and shoulders alone.
2. Make a V-shape with your legs to the sides or forward and back - adding a twist to your waist when you do this.
3. With the legs in the Lotus pose.
4. With your arms on the floor above your head.
5. Making a cycling motion with your legs.
    Come out of this pose as described under the Plough.

5. The Plough

The transition from the Shoulderstand to the Plough can be done in two ways:

1. Lower your back and your legs, held straight, slowly to the floor. Lie briefly in Dead Still.
    Exhale and lift your legs straight upright again, then swing them up over your head until your feet touch the floor beyond your head, so that your upper torso is vertical to the floor.

2. From the Shoulderstand, lower your legs, keeping them straight, over your head until your feet touch the floor beyond your head.

Your arms may rest, either as in the Shoulderstand, if that is necessary, or 1. straight out from the back; 2. over your head pointing to your toes; 3. joined behind your head.

Stay in the Plough for a while, at first less than a minute. Eventually increase the time to three to five minutes, with a maximum of ten minutes.

Concentration: Manipura Chakra at the navel.

The Plough normalizes adrenalin secretion. It is recommended against diabetes and reduces excess weight.

Use it carefully as a beginner; never force yourself into these poses.

Variations:
1. Move on tiptoes as far away from your head as you can, feel your chin touching your chest, then tiptoe back towards your head - back and forth several times.
2. Move on tiptoes from one side to the other as far as you can.
3. Raise one leg vertically, keeping the other on the floor, then the reverse.
4. Grasp your toes and spread your legs as far as possible.
5. Bend your knees as you exhale and draw them in to your ears. Hold this for some time, perhaps with your arms around the backs of your knees.

6. The Reversing pose

Transition from the Plough. Roll up to the Shoulderstand and from there down, so that the root of the hands presses into the waist and supports the hip bone. Keep the legs as vertical as possible. The upper part of the body is at an angle and the hips are resting in the hands. The forearms support the whole lower part of the body and are completely vertical. Stay in it as long as you can or want, if you like twenty minutes.

The Reversing pose preserves youth and vitality, counteracts overweight, prevents the decaying process of the body and improves the metabolism.

Concentration: Vishuddhi Chakra at the throat.

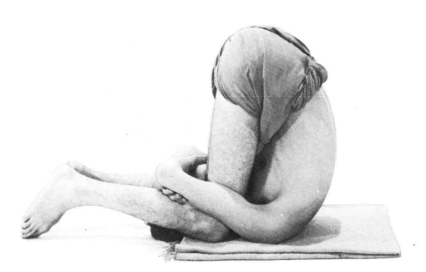

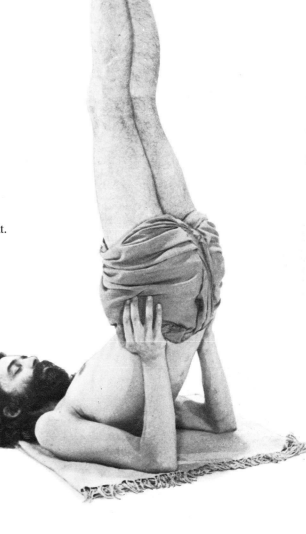

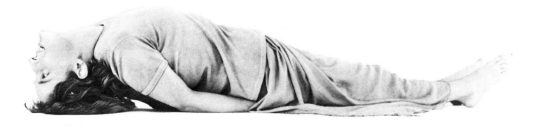

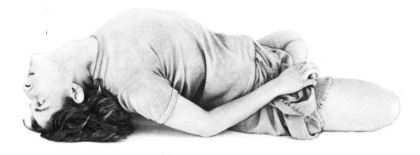

8. The Back Stretch

Dynamic version

1. Lie with your arms at your sides.

2. As you inhale deeply, raise your arms over your head until they touch the floor above your head (brief pause).

3. Hold your breath and sit up, your arms straight over your head.

4. Then lean forward as you exhale and touch your toes. The forehead should touch the knees, if possible.

5. Immediately let your body, without inhaling, roll back to a lying position with your arms sliding by your sides. As you inhale, again lift your arms up beyond your head...

Repeat five times without extra breaths. On the fifth time remain bending forward and breathe normally. Grasp your big toes, with index finger and long finger between the big toe and the next one, your thumbs holding the outer sides of the big toes. This is important, as it influences the nervous currents flowing through Muladhara Chakra.

If you can't reach your big toes, hold your ankles or calves, but keep your legs straight.

7. The Fish

This pose is the counterpose to the three preceding ones. It can be done in two variations, one easy and the other for those who can assume the Lotus pose.

1. Lie in the Dead Still. Place the hands under the buttocks, palms up. Bend the head backward, supporting it on the crown. Push the chest up with the upper part of the body supported by the elbows. Buttocks and legs remain on the floor.

2. Lean back from the Lotus pose until you are resting on the crown. Grasp your feet.

Stay in this pose up to five minutes or as long as you held the Shoulderstand.

Concentration: Manipura Chakra at the navel.

The intestines are stretched and the lungs are expanded. The Fish helps prevent constipation, bronchitis and asthma.

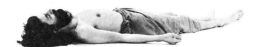

After the Fish pause in Dead Still.

Instruction for the use of Pratyahara
(see also chapter 9)

If you feel pain
or tensions in this pose,
find where the tensions are -
very precisely.
Find the pain! Where is it? How great is it?
How far does it extend?
And then...
Go **into** the pain;
experience it **from within**
as something interesting,
something you don't necessarily need
to be free from.
Go right into the pain,
experience it there.

74

Find the pain's centre.
Mentally touch this place
just where it hurts the most.
Stubbornly hold on to
this place,
this experience.
And if the pain moves,
follow it.
And if you manage
to "touch" the pain,
it will soon
be hard to find.

When tensions are released this way, when
the mind has lost interest in them, then start
observing whether the rest of your body is
relaxed. Is your face relaxed? Feel how your
face is, relax it, from within. Relax the sides
of your throat. Relax your stomach.
Experience your stomach as if it were made
of slowly melting wax.

The classical version
Hold the pose and experience the whole body
at once - a relaxed whole. Feel the body, the
whole body, relaxing.

Or, use your imagination to enhance this
experience of the body resting in itself.
Picture the form of your body sitting in the
pose - as a relaxed whole.

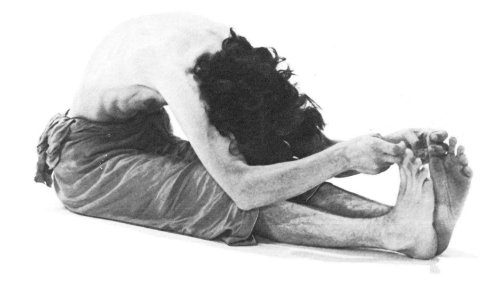

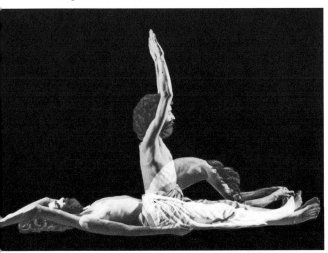

Instruction for concentrating on a chakra
Concentrate at the base of the spine, on
Swadhisthana Chakra as the focal point of
this relaxed body. Stay a long time like this.

Meditating, when coming out of the pose
Let go of your toes, experience the effect of
straightening up coming out of the Back
Stretch. You may now experience a peaceful
feeling spreading through the body. Avoid
unnecessary movements, sit relaxed, but very
still with a straight back and closed eyes.
After a while, focus your attention on the
spine, experience your spinal cord. Move
your consciousness from Muladhara to Ajna
and back, several times, fast or slow.

For more advanced students who are experienced in controlling their breathing
While you are in the pose, exhale completely.
With the vacuum thus created, draw your
diaphragm and stomach upward and
backward towards your spine and contract

your anus and perineum (see Locks, page 82).

Now bend your head even further toward
your knees. Hold the pose as long as you can
without inhaling.

Coming out, first relax the lowest
contraction, then the abdomen and finally:
a. Release your toes and inhale, or
b. Stay in the pose, breathe and stabilize your
breath, then exhale again and repeat the Locks.

There are other variations to this pose, e.g.
holding your toes and ankles with parted legs,
as well as the one described on page 53.

Rules for the Back Stretch: People with disc
trouble should not do this pose at all, or else
only do the dynamic version with the greatest
care. You are the best judge of the way to do
this pose. People who suffer from chronic
constipation should only sit for three minutes.

Pass from this pose to the Abdominal Stretch,
which is the counterpose to the Back Stretch.

9. The Abdominal Stretch

Easy version

Lie on your back. Bend your right knee so that the sole of the foot rests on the floor. Grasp your right ankle and pull that foot back along the outer side of the body resting it beside your hips, either with the toes out or, better, with the foot up alongside the body, sole turned upward. Then carefully move your knee towards the floor using the weight of your legs.

Notice how the front of the thigh is stretched. Relax the shoulders and the front of your throat. Each time you exhale, relax and notice how your knee gets closer and closer to the floor. Focus on the muscles on the front of the thigh.

Then stretch out your leg.

Now bend both knees and pull them up to your chest as a countermove.

Repeat with the left leg.

The classical version

If you can get your knees to the floor then use the following classical variation: Sit in the Diamond pose, with your toes touching and heels out to the sides so that your feet form a "bowl" for the buttocks. Keep your knees close together, if possible. Lean back, rest on your elbows, then on the top of your head and finally let your shoulders and the back of your neck touch the floor. Your knees should still be on the floor (but don't force them) and your palms on your thighs.

Watch your breathing, which should be normal; feel the weight of your shoulders and arms, and if your knees are not there yet, let them get closer and closer to the floor.

Advanced version

Lie in this pose for a long time rather than several short times.

Benefits

The Abdominal Stretch is good for the intestines, which are fully stretched. It stimulates digestion and helps prevent constipation. It stretches the back, especially the small of the back and removes tensions there. Back pains disappear with regular use of the pose. It is also good against sterility and impotence.

Variations:
1. If your knees can't reach the floor you can rest on the top of your head instead of on your shoulders, keeping your hands on your thighs. (If you can't do The Fish, use this variation.)

2. Palms joined on your chest in a "greeting", with shoulders and back touching the floor.

3. Arms raised over your head. This is a good position for your arms in the Abdominal Stretch, as it makes the body stretch even

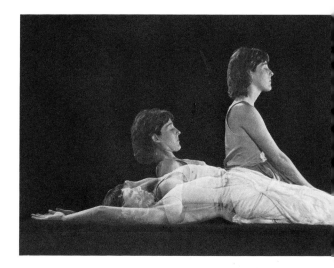

more. This variation is done when your shoulders are touching the floor.

4. Arch your back as far as possible, pushing your stomach up. Rest on your lower legs and the top of your head only. Keep your hands on your thighs.

5. Start with 4. and then with the help of your hands bring your head closer to your feet - by regular use of this exercise it will become possible to touch your feet with your head.

Instruction in body awareness

Think of your stomach, while you are sitting in the pose, feel it, relax it.
Move it gently up and down,
completely relaxing it.

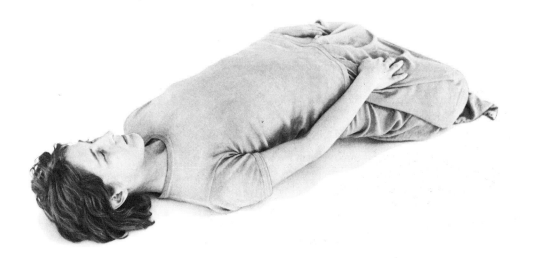

Instruction for the use of Pratyahara

If you find the Abdominal Stretch too difficult, do an easier variation. Or, use Pratyahara as with the Back Stretch - in this pose you may be even more motivated to use it.

If you feel pain
or tension in this pose,
find where the tensions are
exactly.
Find the pain! Where it is?
How great is it?
How far does it extend?
and then...
Go into the pain,
experience it from within
as something interesting,
something you don't necessarily need
to be free from.

Go right into the pain,
experience it there.

Find the pain's centre.
Mentally touch that place
just where it hurts the most.
Stubbornly hold on to
this place,
this experience.

If the pain moves,
follow it.
And if you manage
to "touch" the pain,
it will soon
disappear.

Instruction for concentrating on a chakra

When the stomach is completely relaxed,
bring your attention up
and hold it
at your heart,
in front of your chest,
be aware of this area
around and slightly above
the chest cavity.
Rest in this place.

And after a while
sink backwards
into your chest, towards
your back - to a point
in your spine
at the height of your heart:
Anahata Chakra.
Repeat this several times.

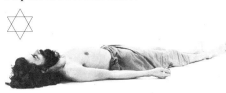

Pause in Dead Still.

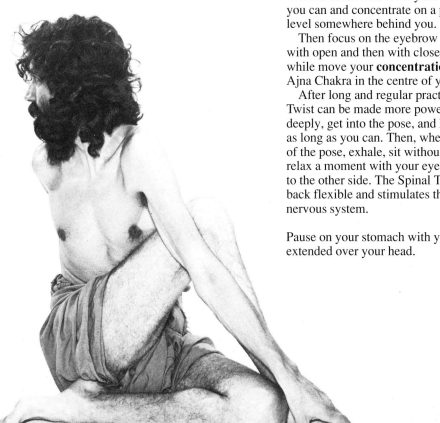

10. The Spinal Twist

1. Sit on the floor. Press your right heel into the groin, so that it rests against your seatbone (if that is too difficult in the beginning, place the foot beside your buttock).
2. Place the left leg on the outer side of the right knee.
3. Twist your body to the left, let the right upper arm touch the outer side of the left thigh and grasp your left foot, so that your fingers bend under the arch from the inner side of the foot. The left arm is stretched behind the back, the fingers touching the right thigh.
4. Look as far back over your left shoulder as you can and concentrate on a point at eye level somewhere behind you.

Then focus on the eyebrow centre, first with open and then with closed eyes. After a while move your **concentration** backward to Ajna Chakra in the centre of your head.

After long and regular practice, the Spinal Twist can be made more powerful: inhale deeply, get into the pose, and hold your breath as long as you can. Then, when you come out of the pose, exhale, sit without moving and relax a moment with your eyes closed. Repeat to the other side. The Spinal Twist makes the back flexible and stimulates the central nervous system.

Pause on your stomach with your arms extended over your head.

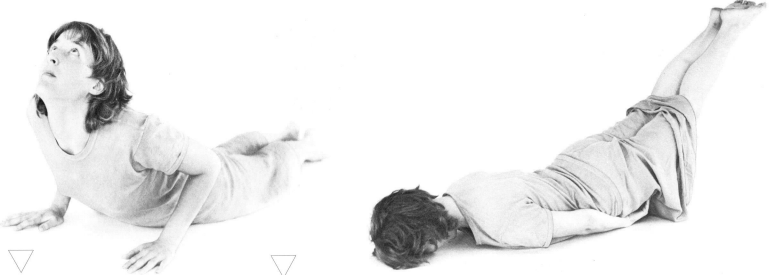

11. The Cobra

1. Lie on your stomach.
2. Put your hands on the floor beside your chest, with your fingers pointing forward.
3. Inhale and slowly raise, first your head, then your shoulders, then your chest, then your stomach - down to the navel. Keep the body below the navel on the floor.
4. Exhale and slowly lower your body to the floor.

While in the Cobra, relax your arms from within. Experience it as if your back alone is supporting the pose - and doing it effortlessly. When experienced, also relax the buttocks.

At first, for a physical effect, go in and out of the pose several times, each time holding the pose briefly. To attain a psychic effect, stay in the Cobra as long as you can.

Concentration: on Vishuddhi Chakra at the throat. This pose makes the spine flexible, is good for the abdomen, can relieve pelvic and menstrual pains, and maybe even cure sciatica and correct disc problems.

Rest for a while on your stomach with your arms extended over your head, but get on with it, don't enjoy the effect of the pose for too long. Do another round or proceed to:

12. The Locust

1. Place your hands, palms up, in under your thighs (or make fists, or interlock your hands, or turn the arms with palms against the floor).
2. Keep your forehead on the floor, inhale and lift your legs as high as you can off the floor, preferably in one swift, sudden movement. Keep your legs there as long as you can. Hold your breath in the pose.

Note: at first you can practise by lifting one leg at a time.

The Locust is most effective for stomach and intestinal diseases. It is good for the abdominal organs, liver, kidneys, pancreas, and it stimulates the appetite. Avoid the pose if you have hernia, ulcers, sores in the alimentary canal, or intestinal tuberculosis.

Concentration: on Vishuddhi Chakra.

Rest a while on your stomach, then go on to:

13. The Bow

1. Bend your knees and hold your ankles.
2. Inhale and stretch your legs so only the abdomen remains on the floor.
3. Hold your breath in the pose as long as possible.

Variations:
1. Rock back and forth in the pose while you hold your breath.
2. Rock to the sides.

The Bow removes superfluous fat. It strengthens the abdominal organs and muscles and makes the spine flexible; it also counteracts constipation and a sluggish liver. It is highly recommended for disc problems. Avoid this pose if you have intestinal sores, ulcers or intestinal tuberculosis.

Concentration: on Vishuddhi Chakra.

Stay in this pose as long as you can. Do it at least three times and after the last time immediately turn over on your back, into Dead Still.

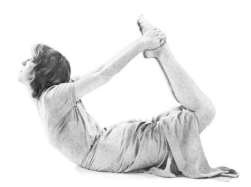

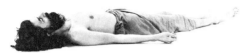

 Pause in Dead Still.

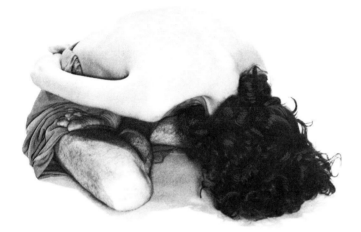

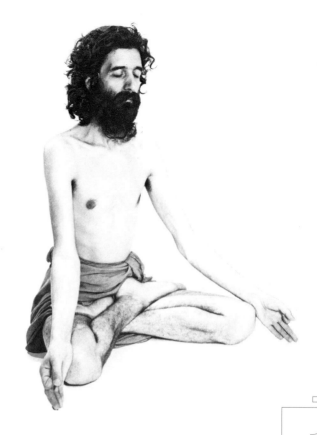

14. The Yoga Attitude

...or harmonizing the energy field of the body.

1. Sit in the Lotus pose.
2. Hold your right wrist with your left hand behind your back.
3. Slowly lean forward as you exhale until your head rests on the floor. Then breathe normally. Relax and feel your body's form and natural breathing. Stay in this position with your eyes closed for three to five minutes.

The Yoga Attitude has a calming and harmonizing effect on the whole body, therefore it is used at the end of the programme. It stimulates the spine and intestines and removes constipation.

Concentration: on Manipura Chakra.

Variation:
Clench your fists, press them against your lower abdomen and lean forward.

Sit still, coming up from the Yoga Attitude.

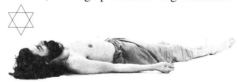

Lie for a while in Dead Still before beginning the breathing exercises (or the Deep Ones page 82).

The Short Programme

Before you take up the long programme of the fourteen exercises described above, start with the shorter one of ten poses in the following order:

1. the Shoulderstand	6. the Locust
2. the Plough	7. the Bow
3. the Fish	8. the Spinal Twist
4. the Back Stretch	9. the Headstand
5. the Cobra	10. Dead Still

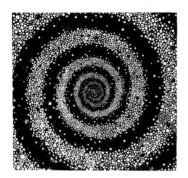

Breathing III

7. The Blacksmith's Bellows 2

Do this cleansing breath when you have mastered its variation on page 49.

1. Sit with your hands resting on your knees. Breathe in and out rapidly and forcefully through both nostrils. Do this twenty times. Your stomach expands when you inhale and contracts when you exhale.

2. Inhale deeply and hold your breath, bend the head forward and lock the throat in the Chin Lock (page 82). Raise your shoulders and support both arms, held straight, on the knees. Pull the sex organs, perineum and anus in and up, at the same time - this is the Root Lock. Hold these two locks, the upper and the lower, as long as you can hold your breath without discomfort (see also page 82).

3. Open the locks by relaxing the Root Lock first and the Chin Lock by raising your head and only then exhale.
 This is one round - do three rounds.
 Note: One round can now be combined

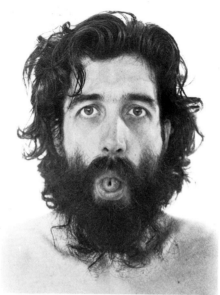

with the Blacksmith's Bellows 1 (page 49). First breathe 20 times through one nostril and hold the breath, then repeat through the other - and finally through both as above.

8. The Cooling Breath

1. Make a tube of your tongue and inhale through that, slowly, making a slight sound.

2. Hold your breath for a while with both locks as in the Blacksmith's Bellows 2.

3. Unlock and exhale through your nose.

The Cooling Breath is done after the other breathing exercises. It is calming, purifies the blood and is an aid against high blood pressure. The norm is nine rounds, but for high blood pressure you can do up to forty-nine rounds. This breath reduces thirst sensation.

Variation:
If you can't roll your tongue, then 1. Clench your teeth and stretch your lips to the corners of your mouth and as far apart as you can, curl your tongue back so the tip touches the soft palate and inhale slowly through your teeth. 2 and 3 are the same as above.

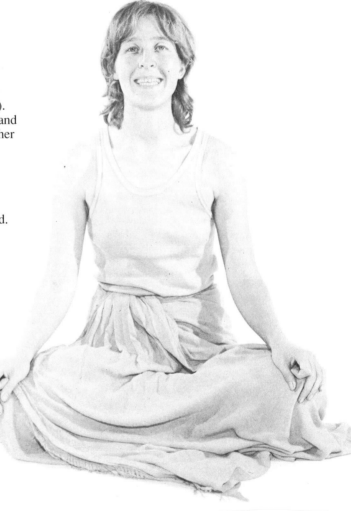

9. The Sun Breath

This is a healing breath, which affects the physical body through the "sun" nostril (see chapter 5 on Hatha Yoga).

The Sun Breath gives an even distribution of psychic energy and levels out the differences between hyper and sub-tensions throughout the body. It has a strong healing effect on all kinds of diseases, from a common cold to blood poisoning and chronic constipation.

1. Close your eyes and relax completely. Sit with your spine straight. Close your left nostril with your right ring finger and inhale through your right nostril; inhale so deeply that you absolutely cannot take in any more air.

2. Close both nostrils - and watch that no air slips out - bend your head into the Chin Lock, pull up the Root Lock. Hold your breath as long as you **possibly** can; then release the Root Lock and the Chin Lock and exhale through your right nostril. This is one sequence; at first do at least three but never more than ten.

10. Alternate Breathing 3

Now we will see how this harmonizing breath is done in its complete form. Its Sanskrit name is *Nadi Shodana*, which means cleansing the energy flows of the body. It has been shown to create a better balance and communication between the two brain halves. My experience is that it removes unwanted states and gives clarity to the mind. It can be a great tool for people who do intellectual and creative work.

For the yogi it is the means to experience the Prana, the psychic energy, and thus to get in touch with the chakras.

Thereby the covering of light disappears
(Patanjali, Yoga Sutras).

You should first master both earlier steps (pages 43 and 49) before you start this. When you inhale count for example to 4, when you hold your breath count to 16, and then exhale to the count of 8. If this number seems too much of a strain, do 3:12:6 - the ratio is always 1:4:2:1:4:2 and it should be carefully observed.

In through the left nostril, hold your breath, out through the right, in through the right, hold your breath, out through the left. When you count, always use the same rhythm, as regular as the slow tick on an old pendulum clock. Here are more advanced counts:
Easy: 12:48:24
Medium: 16:64:32
Advanced: 20:80:40
When you have mastered a number, you can also hold your breath out for the same count after exhaling, before you proceed to a higher number - e.g., in 12, hold 48, out 24, hold 24 - One round is 1:4:2:2:1:4:2:2. Do five rounds.

Note: If you want to do this exercise, you must do it very regularly - observe the instructions scrupulously and do it at the same time every day.

Conclusion

It is best to do breathing exercises after yoga poses and before meditation. If you want to do breathing exercises several times a day, which is only recommended if you do them very regularly, then practise them in the morning after yoga and before breakfast, and in the afternoon a while before the evening meal. For an advanced programme I suggest:

Morning:
The Blacksmith's Bellows, 3 rounds.
The Sun Breath, 3-5 times.
The Cooling Breath, 3-9 times.
Alternate Breathing, 5 rounds.
Meditation with Psychic Breathing, 15-30 minutes (see chapter 11).

Afternoon:
The experience of Spontaneous Breathing (page 43), 10 minutes.
Alternate Breathing, 5 rounds.
Psychic Breathing, 15-30 minutes.

Follow the instructions precisely, observe the few rules (page 43) and do the exercises as regularly as you can for them to have the intended effect.

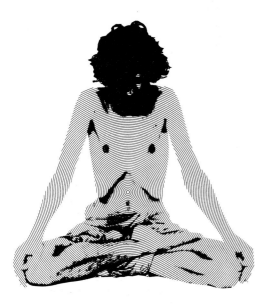

The Deep Ones

This programme contains some deep-working Attitudes (*Mudra*) and also all the Locks (*Bandha*). They can be used separately or together with some of the yoga programmes. The ones on the next page are especially effective when used before meditation.

The Chin Lock
Jalandhara Bandha

Sit in a meditation pose where you can keep your knees on the floor (page 84). The ordinary tailor pose, cross-legged, won't do!

Place your hands on your knees. Close your eyes and relax your whole body. Inhale deeply and hold your breath. Bend your head forward, press your chin against your chest. Straighten your arms, raise your shoulders, and let the body lean a little forward with straight arms and hands pressing lightly on your knees. Hold this pose as long as you can hold your breath. (See the picture on page 81.)

When you come out of the Chin Lock, **first** relax shoulders and arms and undo the lock by raising your head. **Then** exhale slowly.

This exercise can also be done after exhaling. Remember never to breathe in (or out) before the Chin Lock is released and the head is raised. If you cough it means that you are not following this rule.

The Chin Lock produces relaxation throughout body and mind, and relieves the heart by slowing the heart beat. This is achieved on the physical plane by pressing sinus-receptors in the throat area. These receptors ("receivers") respond to blood pressure in the throat artery that supplies blood to the brain. If the pressure is too high, these receptors send impulses to the brain and heart which decreases its activity. If the pressure is too low, the heart rate is quickened. The receptors are sensitive to pressure, and the pressure they are subjected to in the Chin Lock slows down heart activity and creates peace in the mind. The thyroid and the parathyroid are stimulated and their activity is harmonized. These glands, especially the thyroid, affect a great many processes in the human organism, including growth and sexual functions. In this way the entire body benefits from their healthy function.

This is a good exercise for reducing stress, anxiety and anger - and it is a fine preparation for meditation.

The Root Lock
Mula Bandha

If you have prepared for this exercise with the Mare and the Thunderbolt (page 67), it will be quite easy to understand and to do. Sit in a meditation pose with your knees resting firmly on the floor, preferably in the Perfect pose (page 85).

1. Start by pulling in the perineum (the area between the genitals and the anus) - a little pull of just the perineum which is about the size of a big coin. Keep it tense and drawn together for a while, making sure that this contraction does not move forward or backward, concentrating on the area. Then relax it. Just above this, a couple of inches, is the Muladhara Chakra, the root chakra.

2. Pull this contraction upward towards Muladhara Chakra, hold it for some time and then relax it. Do this a few times.

3. Now place your hands on your knees, with your arms straight. Raise your shoulders slightly. Inhale and bend your head forward into the Chin Lock. Then pull up the perineum and hold it as long as you can. This should also result in the contraction of the sex organs and the anus, but the focal point is the perineum and just above it.

First relax the Root Lock, then the Chin Lock and your shoulders and then exhale. Repeat this up to ten times. The Root Lock removes deep-seated tensions and depressions, gives energy, strengthens the lower organs and bowel movements. Do this carefully and thoroughly, preferably under the guidance of a teacher.

The Abdominal Lock
Uddiyana Bandha

Sit in a meditation pose with your knees on the floor and your hands on your knees. Close your eyes and relax completely. Then exhale fully and hold your breath out.

Do the Chin Lock.

Use the vacuum thus created to suck your abdomen upward under the ribs and backward toward the spine. Hold this lock as long as you can without discomfort.

First relax the abdomen, then the Chin Lock and **then** inhale. Repeat the exercise after your breathing has returned to normal.

The exercise can be repeated up to ten times. Most often it is combined with cleansing processes, breathing exercises and forms part of the Great Lock (see below).

Use it only with an empty stomach. Avoid it during pregnancy or if you have ulcers or a serious heart complaint. The entire lower abdomen is strengthened by this exercise and the digestion stimulated and regulated. It can remove constipation and worms, and also counteracts diabetes.

The Great Lock

Maha Bandha

Sit in a meditation pose, preferably the Perfect pose.

Exhale.

Do the Chin Lock.

Do the Abdominal Lock, and the Root Lock.

Focus on the root chakra, Muladhara Chakra, for a few seconds, saying its name mentally: Muladhara.

Then move your concentration to Manipura Chakra, feel it and name it, and after that do the same at Vishuddhi Chakra and then back to Muladhara Chakra. Go on moving from one chakra to the next, naming them for as long as your can hold the breath out. But finish your round with Muladhara.

Finally relax in this order (1) Root Lock; (2) Abdominal Lock; (3) Chin Lock; (4) breathe in and out and repeat the whole sequence - up to seven times. Little by little extend the length of time you hold your breath out, then you will gradually achieve a stronger effect.

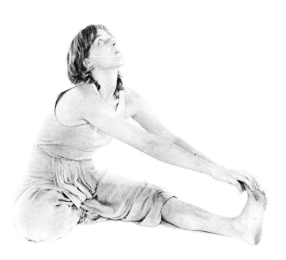

The Great Attitude

Maha Mudra

1. Sit on the floor with your left heel pressed against your perineum and your right leg stretched out in front of your body.

2. Relax completely and inhale deeply.

3. Lean forward and hold the back of your toes with the fingers of both hands. Keep the back straight, especially the small of the back. (If this pose is too hard, use the Perfect pose.)

4. Do the Root Lock and concentrate on the eyebrow centre with your eyes open and the head held back.

5. While holding your breath as long as you can without discomfort, move your consciousness from Muladhara Chakra to Vishuddhi Chakra, then to Ajna Chakra in the middle of your head. Your attention should linger a couple of seconds at each chakra: Muladhara, Vishuddhi, Ajna, Muladhara, Vishuddhi, Ajna, Muladhara. Do this for three rounds.

6. When you can no longer hold your breath, feel Muladhara one last time. Relax the Root Lock, then your eyes, then let go of your toes and slowly exhale through your nose.

7. Repeat the exercise. You begin with three rounds and later the number of rounds can be increased to a maximum of twelve rounds.

8. Change leg positions and do the exercise in the same way with the right heel against your perineum, and then with both legs extended.

The Great Attitude may be used on its own, but it is also very good to practise before meditation since it calms the whole body and mind. It stimulates the flow of psychic energy throughout the body and helps to eliminate depression, lethargy and stomach troubles.

To be as in the Womb

Yoni Mudra

Sit in the Perfect pose (see page 85).

1. Relax and breathe normally.
2. Inhale and hold your breath while you shut

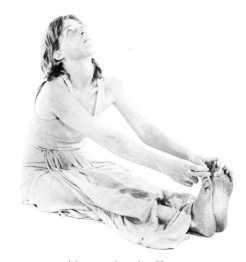

your ears with your thumbs. Keep your eyes closed by resting your index fingers on the lashes of your eyelids without pressure, close your nostrils with both second fingers and your mouth with the ring and little fingers on the upper and lower lips. Then do the Root Lock. Hold this as long as you can hold your breath. Relax from inside. Feel you are in the body. Concentrate on Bindu, the point at the top of the back of your head and listen to the *nada*, inner sounds. This is a more powerful version of exercise 8 in the Ladder (page 68).

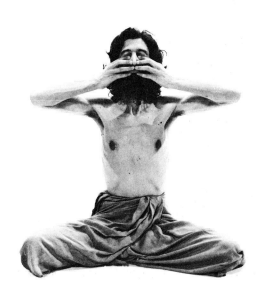

How to sit when you Meditate

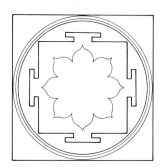

You can sit however you like when you meditate, as long as your body does not disturb you. You can sit in an easy chair, on an office chair, on a straight-backed chair or in a deck chair. In that way you may go further than if you sit and suffer in a difficult position with sore knees and back. But if you want to go deep and experience meditation fully, then you must sit **completely** still during the whole meditation - i.e. no movement - and so you may prefer a straight-backed chair, where you sit upright with your hands resting on your knees, or a yoga meditation pose. Find out for yourself and test the different possibilities.

A real meditation pose may require training, but is a must once you want to use a meditation which works with your energy. Train by using the Pre-meditation poses on page 38. And when your body does not disturb you any more, use the real meditation poses. Until then, continue meditating on a chair.

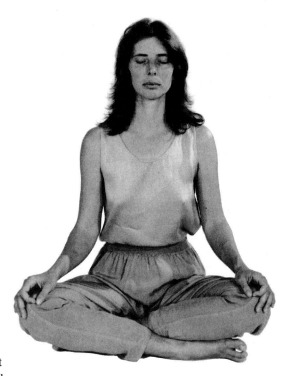

1. The Easy pose

The ordinary Tailor's pose, or sitting cross-legged, is not really a meditation pose, although some people use it as such. If you must use it, at least keep your back straight and place one foot under each thigh. Rest your hands on your knees, hold your head, neck and spine straight.

I recommend you leave this pose as soon as you have learnt one of the following.

2. The Diamond pose

Vajrasana. This very fine pose is described in Loosening the Knots (page 58).

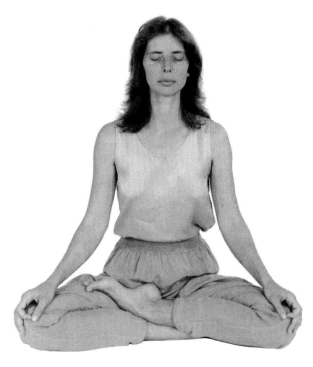

3. Half Lotus

Ardha Padmasana

Bend one leg and place that foot against your thigh. The other foot is placed on top of the opposite thigh with the sole facing up. Keep your knees on the floor and your spine straight. Occasionally alternate the foot that is uppermost, thus training the body for the Lotus pose.

Siddha Yoni Asana, for women:

Sit with your legs straight. Bend one leg and place the sole tight against your thigh next to the groin so that your heel presses against the vagina. Bend your other leg and place that foot with the heel uppermost over the pubic bone in towards the body with your toes between the calf muscle and the thigh. Straighten your back and rest your hands on your knees.

This pose has just recently been made public by Swami Satyananda, who brings it to us from the secret tradition. Siddha Yoni Asana is best practised without underclothes.

Both variations of the pose may be more easily done by placing a little cushion or folded blanket under your buttocks, so that they are slightly raised in relation to your feet.

This pose should be avoided if you have sciatica or inflammation of the sexual organs.

You can sit still for a long time in this pose. It has a strong and calming effect on the whole nervous system. It gives control over sexual impulses and energies that flow to the head, whether you want to use these energies for meditation, sexual pleasure or the development of your concentration.

5. The Lotus pose

Padmasana

Sit with straight legs. Bend one leg and rest that foot above the other thigh with the sole facing up and heel close to the lower abdomen. Then place the other foot similarly on the opposite thigh. Before trying this pose you should have practised the Pre-meditation poses. Don't force your body.

This pose gives the body a stable stance during meditation - and it harmonizes the body's energy flow. It strengthens the lower abdomen, improves digestion and helps prevent emotional, nervous and physical troubles. In medical research, the Lotus pose has been shown to improve the fitness or general condition of the body.

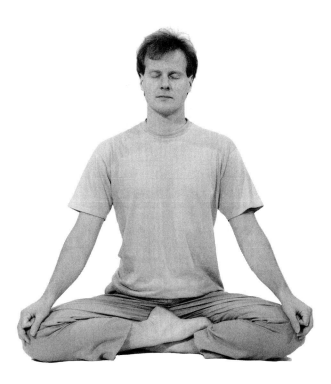

4. The Perfect pose

Siddhasana, for men:

Place one heel against the perineum with the knee touching the floor. You may have to lift the body a little to almost sit on the heel. Then place the other heel in against the body right above the genitals, lightly touching the pubis (just above the penis). Lower the knee to the floor and lock the pose by inserting the toes of the upper foot down into the fold between thigh and calf. Some people can also pull up the toes of the lower foot between the other thigh and calf. Place your hands on your knees.

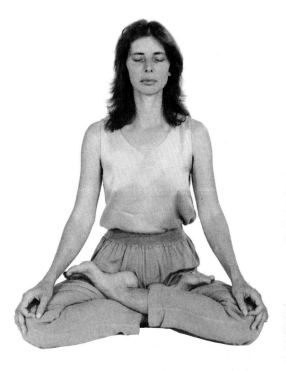

6. Position of the Hands

1."The attitude of awareness", and 2."the attitude of intuition". Bend your index finger and place it against the inner side of your thumb, keeping the other three fingers straight.
1. Palms facing forward, rest the back of your hands on your knees, see page 79 and 111, or:
2. Palms down, place your hands on your knees.

Through yoga and meditation, the body and mind adjust to increasingly subtle states; it is therefore important how the nerve impulses and energy currents are flowing. These "attitudes" influence the energy, giving greater calm to the hands - and enabling you to sit still for longer periods.

Chapter 7

The Tantric Sexual Act

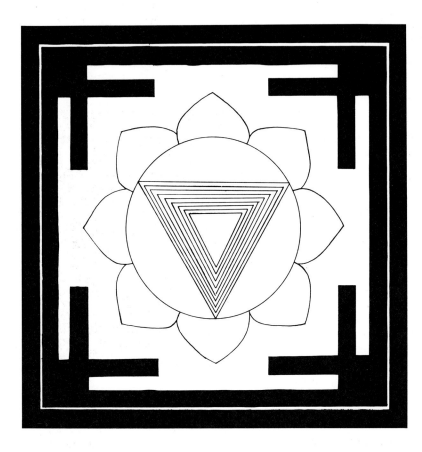

What you are about to discover in this chapter is a ritual of great potential, a process to capture the mind and lead you to greater freedom. To some people, the mere existence of the Tantric Sexual Act is quite revolutionary if not disturbing even today, as it also was in India in former times. And many are the stories that have been told of the Tantrics, based on people's imagination rather than on insight and experience.

Of course anyone may interpret the ritual described here the way he or she wants - psychoanalysis would say that here you are getting in contact with what is archetypically and fundamentally human, the libido.

However, with a sceptical, "inquiring" attitude or with any other reservation, you will not be able to reach into the process - in the act you must be able to let go fully.

To profit from this chapter, it is necessary to have read this book and experienced its exercises.

The sexual challenge

To say the least, sex plays a very important role in our cultures. And why shouldn't it? Sexuality is one of the strongest forces in the human being. And yet we have difficulty in realizing and accepting this need. We tend to look away as if it were something alien or animal. We even become intolerant of ourselves and of others. We tend to underplay sex or else we let it dominate our lives.

It is possible to relate to sex in a natural, accepting way, to experience it as an urge or force in itself, one we all share - and then live with it consciously, using it or transforming it in different ways.

In Tantra and yoga, we find different suggestions for sexual behaviour. Among other things, Tantra is known as "the sexual yoga". It is true that the Tantric science includes this subject but, because of the great immediacy of sexuality, to some people Tantra seems concerned with this area exclusively.

This chapter is for those with a normal sex life, those who have problems with it, and those who view the sexual act as something meaningful and elevating.

By the mere drinking of wine, without initiation, a human being does not become enlightened; only after being fully initiated can a person be called a master.

(Mahanirvana Tantra)

For the Tantric, it is not a matter of avoiding sex by either becoming frantic about it or by suppressing it. To take part in the sexual ritual is a highly conscious approach.

The Tantric Asana unite the spirit and matter and enable a person to attain full self-realization - this effect is a transformation of consciousness. Tantric Yoga accepts this world as Purusha (Man) *and Prakriti* (Woman) *and makes self-realization possible; they pursue their union through deepening and making two into one (two-ness transformed into Oneness).*

From the Tantric viewpoint the perfect human is the melting together of man and woman in the Self - so that the individual consciousness merges into a shared consciousness. This state is called Ananda, eternal bliss, the highest joy.

(Ajit Mookerjee)

Impotence, frigidity and anxiety are removed through the purifying and relaxing effect of yogic exercises and meditation. The experience gained through these practices has prepared you for the sexual meditation - your increased sensitivity and your ability to experience with great intensity will be needed when you place yourself together with one or more in the circle. You should be so securely resting in yourself that neither resistance, fear nor embarrassment will hinder your heightened awareness and your openness to your partner.

In the days before the ritual itself it is a good idea to abstain from sex in order to build up as strong a drive as possible. The drive is the whole foundation for the transformation of consciousness. Without urge, there is no energy, no interest, no transformation.

In the three Ages this rite was a great secret; men then used to perform it in all secrecy, and thus attained liberation. When the Age of Kali prevails, the devotees should declare themselves as such, and whether in the night or the day, should openly be initiated.

(Mahanirvana Tantra)

Preparation

Contact between the sexes is experienced in so many ways from the glance of an eye to intercourse.

Everything preceding the act itself is dedicated to raising consciousness and relieving tensions.

1. The room where the ritual will take place is cleaned. Incense should burn there all the time. Your nose and olfactory organs are connected by nerves and subtle psychic currents to the Muladhara Chakra where the Kundalini lies coiled. When your sense of smell is affected, your awareness will be heightened and you will become more sensitive. See also chapter 8.

2. Prepare the food and flowers to be used during the ritual. The meal consists of four different ingredients and the room should be decorated with flowers:

Wine
Wine symbolizes the intoxicating experience of the richness of consciousness attained through yoga. (If you prefer not to use alcohol, substitute coconut milk.)

Meat
Meat symbolizes everything that I am, all that I do and experience - I stand by this: all is part of my being. (If you do not eat meat, substitute garlic, ginger, salt, sesame seeds or wheat.)

Fish
Fish symbolizes a state in which I experience all, the whole universe, pleasure and pain, as myself. "I am all this. I contain all contradictions." (If you do not eat fish, use radishes.)

Roasted cereals
They symbolize that I give up identifying myself with fear and inhibitions.

Flowers
Flowers symbolize the intercourse which in turn symbolizes the primal force (the female, energy and matter) rising to the highest chakra, Sahasrara, uniting there with consciousness, the male.

3. You should bathe together. This relaxes and envigorates, preparing both of you to meet your "divine partner". The *Shakti* (the woman who symbolizes all women) is rubbed with scented oils and perfumes. Various oils may be rubbed on different parts of the body; for example musk oil around the mount of Venus.

There is also a way to massage the spine of your partner. Starting at the base of the spine, press your thumbs lightly on either side of the protruding centre bone. Rub the thumbs alternately back and forth in small movements, working your way slowly up the spine. The area of Sushumna, Ida and Pingala will be freed of tensions and sensitized.

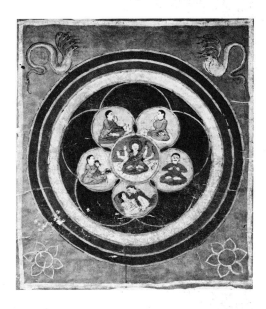

Becoming Attuned...

The room has been decorated with flowers, food is laid out and the wine decanted, incense glows, candles burn or better still an oil lamp with oil that creates a special red light.

The next step of this elevated event is to initiate and cleanse the room and the house, sprinkling water and using mantras. Normally long verses of mantras are used; this part of the ritual can be rich and complex in order to constantly keep the mind occupied (tensions then find no place) and heightened.

Here I have chosen the use of the mantra *Am, Hrim, Krom, Hamsah, So-Ham* which is said aloud and repeated eleven times: in the room, to those present, to the food, to the wine, to the four corners of the world, and to what is above and below. Have a small bowl of water in front of you, dip your fingers into it and sprinkle the water as above saying the mantra *Swaha* (I burn it - I offer it). Also dip some flowers in the water and throw them on the food - *Swaha* - on the wine - *Swaha* - on those present - *Swaha*...

This practice should go on so long and thoroughly that you become completely absorbed, so that you give yourself seriously and without reservation.

With her finger dipped in red powder mixed with a little soapy water and oil, Shakti places a red mark on the eyebrow centre of those present. She is given a mark too. This symbolizes the level of concentration and ability to participate that is reached through Ajna Chakra in the centre of the head. If Ajna Chakra is awakened, you will participate in this act without tension, without being blocked by emotions of shame or frivolity.

Yoga and Meditation

Do the programme of mudras called the Ladder (page 66) or the Deep Ones (page 82). Use the mantra *So-Ham* with Psychic Breathing (page 111) or with normal breathing (or use your own mantra). Meditate a while on *So-Ham, So* as you inhale and *Ham* as you exhale.

Begin by meditating on your body. Then meditate for a while on your breathing and repeat the mantra *Am, Hrim, Krom, Hamsah, So-Ham*. Experience your body as light - imagine that your body is made of pure light and that this light destroys every single fear in you, every inhibition and all hatred. Observe

how this prepares you for the cosmic act which is experienced as the union of the female force and the male consciousness. Experience a strengthening and cleansing flow of light filling your whole body and your breathing.

The Ritual

If more people are present one is appointed the guru and leads the ritual. He should dip his second finger in the water and draw a

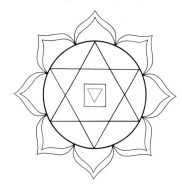

triangle pointing down ▽ on the floor where you are sitting and then over it draw a triangle pointing up △ . And then in the centre of both triangles, the centre of that six-pointed star, a smaller square □ is drawn and in the square another triangle standing on its point ▽ .

The two triangles symbolize respectively the female ▽ and the male △ part of the universe. The square ▽ symbolizes the foundation from which the force is awakened and raised. The force is symbolized by the last triangle. A circle is drawn around both triangles touching all six points - this symbolizes eternity. Then eight lotus petals

are drawn outside the circle - symbolizing infinity.

Finally, the conclusion of the invocation: Shakti consecrates the wine using the mantra *Swaha*, flowers and water. She pours the wine for all present. The wine should be strong enough to have a freeing effect on the mind, but don't drink so much that you cannot keep your awareness clear.

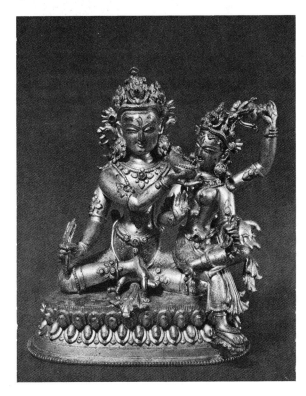

Now the man sits in a meditation pose (if possible). The woman sits on his left thigh and they give each other first the wine and then the food; they feed each other. If you find this pose too difficult, you could also sit beside each other, the woman to the left of the man.

As scents affect Muladhara Chakra (the root chakra), Swadhisthana Chakra (the sexual chakra) is affected by eating and drinking. This increases energy, desire and sensitivity (chapter 8).

The Act

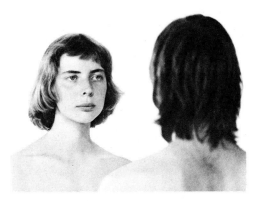

This exercise - or more accurately this act - is preparatory in relation to the pose itself; it gives insight and experience. Sit facing your partner and look into each other's eyes. You are completely naked and you sit facing each other as two people, as man and woman, and experience each other's sex and desire. You recognize each other, you take part in a universal event, two divine people together with the universe.

Meditate on each other, experience each other with desire and joy. If you smile self-consciously or if you tense your facial muscles or body, return to a relaxed natural state each time. Get back into the play and the seriousness of what you are doing again and again. If limiting thoughts surface - whatever happens, accept it briefly - then turn back to the experience of each other. Naked you face each other, open and sensitive, experiencing each other's body, each other's eyes, and the many masks that appear as you concentrate on a face - let it all come and go. Uninterrupted and for a long time, go on experiencing your divine partner. You don't have to demand or explain or excuse anything. You do not have to accomplish anything - be - experience - enjoy!

Then proceed with the intercourse. This can be done in two ways, **either** in the following way, **or** in the Tantric poses.

Give yourself freely to the intercourse with

joy and as unrestrained as gods. Or, as if a god and goddess have been invited into your bodies, pass on all happiness and enjoyment to them, and also every doubt and inhibition that might occur. Everything is passed on right away - everything, good or bad, is ceaselessly passed on, accepted and released. Everything is part of the universe, neither enjoyment nor suffering is our individual property - all that we do is devotion and in this devotion we live.

In the Tantric poses, you assume a yogic sexual position. You don't do this mechanically or by getting up and then lying down again. Rather, you do it without losing contact with each other even for an instant, so that without interrupting the play you unite pleasurably and sensually. There are several positions:

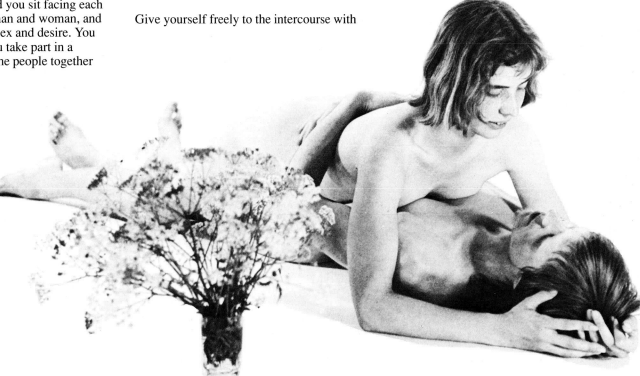

The Poses

1. The man sits in a meditation pose and the woman sits down on the man bending her legs around the man's waist and hips, so that her feet are crossed behind his buttocks.

2. Same as 1, but instead of the woman crossing her legs behind him, she raises them, while the man keeps his arms under her knees and embraces her round her waist and small of the back.

3. The man lies on his back and the woman squats on him.

4. The woman starts by sitting as in 3 then she lies back between his legs, extending her legs along his body.

5. Standing. The man stands on the floor supporting the woman, while she holds on to him with her legs and arms around him.

6. The woman lies straight on top of the man.

There are many variations. However the back must be straight or held as in a yoga pose. Remain motionless in the pose, while you

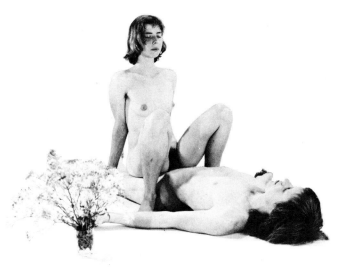

experience each other physically and psychically. Together you enter into an unbroken sexual meditation. You are **motionless**. The experience of psychic and universal union can occur at any time and when it occurs remain in it as long as it is at its height, then end it. The shortest time for a pose may have to be a little over half an hour for any real change or transformation to take place.

You need not be overly concerned with the body. This is not a performance! Let the Shakti in your partner lead and inspire you. Just give and receive. The way you sense each other physically and psychically is what matters. You do not have to strive for any "normal" orgasm or release - let the experience of each other, of a common energy field and a shared consciousness, transform you. Think of the experiences you have had in other meditations: of your whole body, of your breath, of your energy. Trust that you are doing the right thing. This sketch can only be a starting point. Let the sexual energy grow and fill your bodies.

Don't speculate beforehand about how the meditation will work out. Expectations might prevent you from being open to whatever comes by itself. That is not worth the risk.

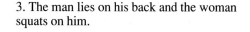

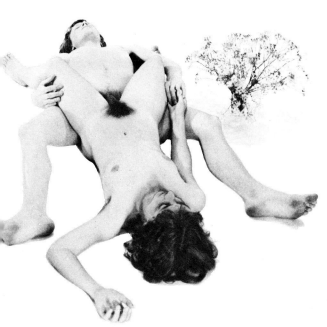

There are sixty-four different sexual yoga poses and each pose gives a different experience; the energy flows differently and, just as in other yoga poses which you have experienced, each pose has its own effect.

People change, even those you "know". Experiences differ. Do you know in advance how everything will be? Take an initiative, decide which way you want to go. But once you have chosen the direction, let it happen. Receive and be surprised.

The sixty-four poses symbolize freedom from expectations. Each time you can do it in a new way. You can also afford to use the same pose. It's up to you.

A free Act...

If you do not tell others about your experiences in yoga and meditation, or do not hold on to your experiences as if you intend to repeat them, you increase your ability to experience everything always as if it were for the first time. Then it doesn't matter whether you're having new experiences or not.

Get used to the ritual, do it many times - gradually you will master it and benefit from

it fully. It may not happen right away and not if you are in a hurry. Only when you feel at ease with it, and can play without straining, will the deeper effect come about.

A ritual symbolizes a free action. It has a set course to ensure the intended transformation. But whether or not you are free, and whether you gain from these methods, depends on you.

Besides the ritual done by a couple, there is a shared ritual of several couples sitting together in a circle. The first parts of the act, for example the bath (comparable to a sauna) and the ritual, are performed all together. The woman chosen to be the Shakti symbolizes the energy for all present in the circle and is honoured as such. She distributes the wine and food and thus initiates the ritual. A guru performs the ritual of mantras and gives instruction concerning the meditation and the course of action. For the intercourse itself, the different poses, each couple sits in a big circle called a *Chakra*. The feast or ritual, the rite of raising the consciousness, is called the *Puja - Chakra Puja*.

Meditation with others generates a powerful energy field, and gives support to every person sharing it. There are different variations of these Pujas: In *Bhairavi Chakra* each has chosen a partner in advance, e.g. married people or those together in a relationship. In *Yogini Chakra* you freely and spontaneously choose partners, and here the partner is experienced as a completely free, independent individual.

A *Chakra* may be performed in different ways. What is essential is that you are receptive to its potential.

I have seen a Tantric manuscript from Bengal which states that these rituals originated in the North, "Thule, which is Scandinavia and those parts north of these". If you have experienced this ritual, you may recognize a hint of it in ancient stone carvings or other ancient historical sources. Of course, it doesn't matter whether it is Indian or Scandinavian: rather it is a common human

event. The form of the ritual is gradually shaped by those who perform it - the tradition is something living and creative.

To elevate the intercourse to a ritual, to a heightened act and a meditation, is so meaningful that it can have profound and liberating effects in our lives. Something often performed unconsciously, mechanically and shamefully, becomes an experience that not only frees you from sexual inhibitions but expands your consciousness in a way that only deep meditation can achieve. It becomes a beautiful and central act in human society.

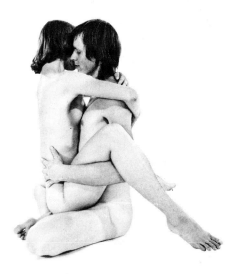

Whatever you do -
do it with inspiration
do it so that you do not lose your energy
do it wholly and fully
with the help of yoga
without shame or fear
freely
and take with you
this freedom and happiness
make it a part of your everyday.

Chapter 8
The Chakras and Kundalini Yoga

The Sensitivity, the Power and the Experience

In the spinal cord connected with the central nervous system, there are what in Tantric science is called the *chakras*.

The meeting with the chakras in Kundalini Yoga happens when we experience the energy as something accessible. When we can accept all the roles that this energy plays and dances for us, then we start to remember and become conscious of the song and dance in ourselves.

On the mental plane, this results in you getting to know yourself, your limitations and capacities. You discover what is behind your personality so you can use it and work with it in quite another way than by living on preconceptions, hopes and dreams.

This is about the fundamental powers in man, the way to experience these forces as something in itself: I am not angry, depressed or excited, but I experience underlying states of energy that I can make use of, transform and express. It gives me insight and a deeper knowledge of what I can do and what I am.

The chakras play an important part in the understanding of how the body's psychosomatic balance can be consciously influenced, that is, the ability to control normally unconscious bodily functions (autonomic processes beyond the will and therefore beyond conscious control). The digestive process can be regulated consciously and there are numerous accounts of yogis decreasing their heart activity to a minimum, so that only very sensitive instruments can register that they are alive at all.

In Kundalini Yoga, we talk of "awakening" these chakras, of the distinct areas of consciousness they cover, and of their abilities.

By now you may have experienced how the **classical yoga poses** balance the chakras in a most essential way. We concentrate primarily on the front of the body in the *contact area* of the chakra, loosening tensions. When the area is awakened and you become sensitive to its energy, you move back with your awareness or feeling to the actual chakra, a smaller area in the spine. When a spinal chakra is affected, it in turn has an effect on a corresponding centre in the brain, which is activated, or made conscious. In this way, gradually, the 80-90 per cent of the brain that is usually dormant is reclaimed. The **Mudras** and **Bandhas** (pages 66 and 82) also influence the chakras, harmonizing their areas by removing any limitation that might have occurred in the energy field of the chakra and thus in your general state and the total form of your energy. In *Yoga Nidra* relaxation and in meditation, the chakras are reached through symbols, mantras (page 95) and yantras (see on page 94). In **meditation**, you gain insight into what they really are: "whirls" or "corridors", penetrating your being, dimensions where body, mind, energy and the innermost part of you communicate.

Through each chakra you access with greater awareness your own deeper emotions and thoughts, and also the signals of the world around you. From your spine, so to speak, you observe the play of energy in the front of your body, and feel how your personality responds to everything, conscious or unconscious.

Chakra means wheel in Sanskrit. Today this knowledge reaches us from the yoga tradition. In early times in Europe, chakras were known to the alchemists, in Israel by the Kabbalists, in Egypt by the Dervishes, in Greenland and Canada by the Inuits and in North America by the Hopi nation. The Hopis are said to be one of the oldest unbroken cultures in the world. From their mythology I have chosen this:

Palöngawhoya, travelling throughout the world, sounded out his call as he was bidden. All the vibratory centers along the earth's axis from pole to pole resounded his call; the earth trembled; the universe quivered in tune. Thus he made the whole world an instrument of sound, and sound an instrument for carrying messages, resounding praise to the Creator of all...

The living body of man and the living body of the earth were constructed in the same way. Through each ran an axis, man's axis being the backbone, the vertebral column, which controlled the equilibrium of his movements and his functions. Along this axis were several vibratory centers which echoed the primordial sound of life throughout the universe or sounded a warning if anything went wrong.

The first of these in man lay at the top of the head. Here, when he was born, was the soft spot, kopavi, the "open door" through

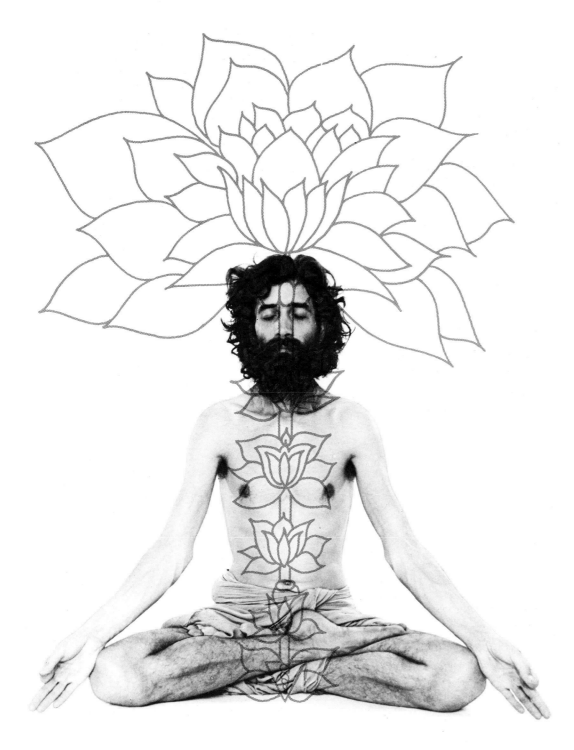

which he received his life and communicated with his Creator...

Just below it lay the second center, it enabled man to think about his actions and work on this earth. But the more he understood that his work and actions should conform to the plan of the Creator, the more clearly he understood that the real function ...was carrying out the plan of the Creation.

The third center lay in the throat... This primordial sound, as that coming from the vibratory centers of the body of the earth, was attuned to the universal vibration of all Creation. New and diverse sounds were given forth by these vocal organs in the forms of speech and song, their secondary function for man on this earth. But as he came to understand its primary function, he used this center to speak and sing praises to the Creator.

The forth center was the heart. It too was a vibrating organ, pulsing with the vibration of life itself. In his heart man felt the good of life, its sincere purpose. He was of One Heart. But there were those who permitted evil feelings to enter. They were said to be of Two Hearts.

The last of man's important centers lay under his navel ... it was the throne in man of the Creator himself. From it he directed all the functions of man.

(F. Waters, Book of the Hopi)

Training

The discovery of yourself cannot be prescribed in any one set way; the teaching and the guidance are both general and highly individual. But in order to avoid confusion it pays to stay with one teaching, one tradition.

To distinguish between what is real and unreal is as difficult as separating milk from water in a mixture of both, and is one of the key issues of yoga. What is imagined about the chakras today, and through hypnosis made to appear as genuine experiences, only hinders one in reaching the real potential of the chakras. You will find people who attach a scale of values to the different chakras; you might as well give different values to your senses, that one eye is better or "higher" than the other.

93

We have seen how yoga can help us reach these areas. But other guidance may also be useful. In case of a radical awakening, for instance, it is necessary to keep a fixed diet. A teacher may be needed, not a lofty person on a throne but a craftsman who knows his trade - as my guru said: "To teach is like living on roses." He/she must be ready to involve you and him/herself in the battle of seeing through illusions - false identifications on which we base our lives and become chained.

Behind everything we experience there is psychic energy. How you perceive it depends on your preconceptions, wishes and problems, that is, on your background and character.

If a chakra is being charged, at first you may not experience it as pure energy, but associate it with thoughts bound in the subconscious or as a tense state; or as some do, you may make the mistake of blaming others for good or bad vibrations. The realization that such a conclusion was your mind attempting to avoid the intense experience of awareness and energy will give you detachment and relaxation.

There are several possibilities as to how to live when you get into advanced yoga: sex or total abstinence may be seen as two extremes from this viewpoint. Celibacy is rather an economical way of life, preserving intensity, energy and oneness, than an absolute prohibition. Energy is lost in many ways and is also gained in many ways, but if you have never built up real energy, then you have no idea of what can be lost. Sexual economy is directed by the brain not the sex organs: energy is not tapped by the release of fluids that have already been accumulated - let it go if it has changed into chemicals that upset your clarity. There is no **one** way, and this has nothing to do with ideals. A person without sexual blocks undoubtedly has more energy than one who is blocked by fear or moral scruples.

"Creative" limiting of oneself is like creating a laser beam that can focus its energy particles and reach anywhere, any distance. An ordinary searchlight diffuses its beam and has a limited effect. An integrated way of living covers more than mere sexual abstinence.

But remember: this is not suicide - this is a matter of intensifying life, and you want it to last: don't stifle yourself, but engage yourself as you want to and can.

The Inner Action
Transformation of energy
The basic method here is Pratyahara (see chapter 9). You saturate the mind with whatever you are experiencing and accept the experience as it is. Let it be, and stay with it, until the mind lets go of it or a transformation occurs. When you are dependent upon attraction and repulsion - no matter whether you call it love or hate, it is basically the same energy - you are holding back. If the energy is to be channelled or transformed and to gain fullness, then you must let go. No matter what the form of the power you meet, experience it and abandon all preconceptions you may have - become one with the fullness of the energy.

Concentrate on whatever state arises in your body and mind, hold on to that experience, enter it, let it fill your mind, let it be just the way it is and relax with it.

In this way different states may be experienced and transformed in relation to the chakras. This is for you to test:

1. Sexual desire
When you feel or evoke sexual desire in your body, let it be there, go with your whole consciousness to the part of the body it comes from and experience how it affects the whole body. While you hold on to that experience, see it as an expression of the underlying energy of the universe. Become one with it, experience it and let it unfold.

You will experience this transformation as a strong and luminous feeling that will fill you fully - mind and body.

2. Apathy or sleepiness
If, for example during meditation, you experience drowsiness (this is natural at first with certain forms of meditation) then observe this sleepiness. Don't disturb it. Feel

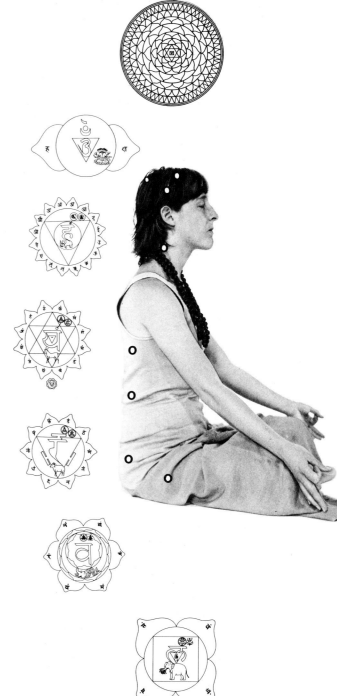

The different chakras are not physical organs. They are areas and points where psychic energy and bodily functions merge.

Name, meaning and number of petals	Area in the body	Physiology	Psychic symbol	Element or quality, sensory experience, organ, yantra colour	Mantra
Sahasrara, the 1000-petal lotus	Whole skull and brain	Pituitary gland	Red 1000-petal lotus on top of the head	Red	All
Bindu, the point or nectar drop	At the top of the back of the head	Vision centre in brain	A crescent moon and a starry night	Tension-dissolving inner sound-space. Light yellow	Nada sound
Ajna, command or control chakra. 2-petal lotus	In the centre of the head behind the eyebrow centre	Plexus cavernosus, pineal gland	A state of absorbtion, a golden egg	The mind. Grey	OM
Vishuddhi, the purification chakra. 16-petal lotus	In the throat, contact area in the front and chakra in the spinal cord	Pharyngeal plexus, larynx, thyroid gland	Nectar drops and the experience of cold	Ether, inner space. Hearing, ears, larynx. Violet	HAM
Anahata, the unbroken sound. 12-petal lotus	Contact, front of the heart, chakra in the spinal cord	Cardiac plexus, thymus gland	A little flame from a small candle or oil lamp	Air. Touch, perception, skin, hands. Dark blue	YAM
Manipura, the jewel's abode. 10-petal lotus	Contact at the navel, chakra in the spinal cord	Solar plexus, pancreas	A golden lotus or water lilly	Fire. Sight, eyes, feet. Gold	RAM
Swadhisthana, one's own place. 6-petal lotus	Contact at the pubis, chakra, base of the spine	Pelvic plexuses, ovaries or testes, adrenal glands	A state of unconsciousness or self-forgetfulness	Water. Taste, tongue, sex organs, kidneys, metabolism. Black	VAM
Muladhara, the fundamental root chakra. 4-petal lotus	Above the perineum between the anus and the sex organs	Coccygeal plexus	Inverted red triangle, inside it an oval form with a snake coiled three and a half times	Earth. Sense of smell, nose, rectum. Yellow	LAM

it in relation to the body, be aware that you can "see" or "notice" sleepiness. Then go into the sleepiness, feel how it affects you, grasp it like an object. If you do this thoroughly and long enough, here you will also experience a change that separates you from the sleepiness and you will experience yourself behind it all.

3. This also applies to anxiety, nervousness, frigidity and stress. You can experience a nervous state in your stomach in this way. Observe how different states affect you. Let it happen - stay with the experience, relax in it, let it be. You can also do this with:
4. jealousy;
5. anger;
6. indecisiveness, indifference and boredom;
7. hate, love, grief, disappointment;
8. enthusiasm, delight;
9. understanding, concentration.

Experience them all in the same way in relation to yourself. If your sensitivity has increased by the use of yoga, breathing exercises and meditation, then learn this process and repeat it over and over, and you will achieve an insight into the chakras and Kundalini Yoga that no theory can give.

The movement of Energy and the cleansing of Chakras

One fine day you will sense the energy that flows and vibrates in the different chakras and in your back. Then you can cause the force to flow from Sahasrara to Muladhara and up from Muladhara through Sahasrara.
This takes training;
it takes time
maturing
cleansing -
and again
from Sahasrara to Muladhara
from Muladhara to Sahasrara
from Manipura to Sahasrara
from Sahasrara to Manipura
from Anahata to Manipura
from Manipura to Anahata.
Be conscious that powerful energy and vibrations should not be avoided. (Remember energy is energy, pure and simple, not good or bad vibrations.) When you experience, for example, the force in Manipura, stay there and contact it; go into it and experience it.
From Vishuddhi to Anahata
from Manipura to Sahasrara

and home again
to Swadhisthana
from Swadhisthana
to Ajna
to Nada in Bindu
to Sahasrara
and around again
down and up
through the psychic passages
in the spinal cord.
If you let a chakra open, accept that one chakra and just work with that, let any tension vibrate away. Later go on to other chakras. Step by step get to know yourself. Remember it doesn't matter which chakra you choose - they are not arranged in order of value. When deep in meditation, experience the psychic symbols related to the different chakras.

The use of Capability

This begins with work and relaxation: you encounter, grasp and let go of subconscious tensions. Inner psychic processes become clear. It leads to knowledge of the interrelatedness of everything - the ability to enter into and adapt to any circumstance whatsoever.

Part Three

The Senses and the Mind

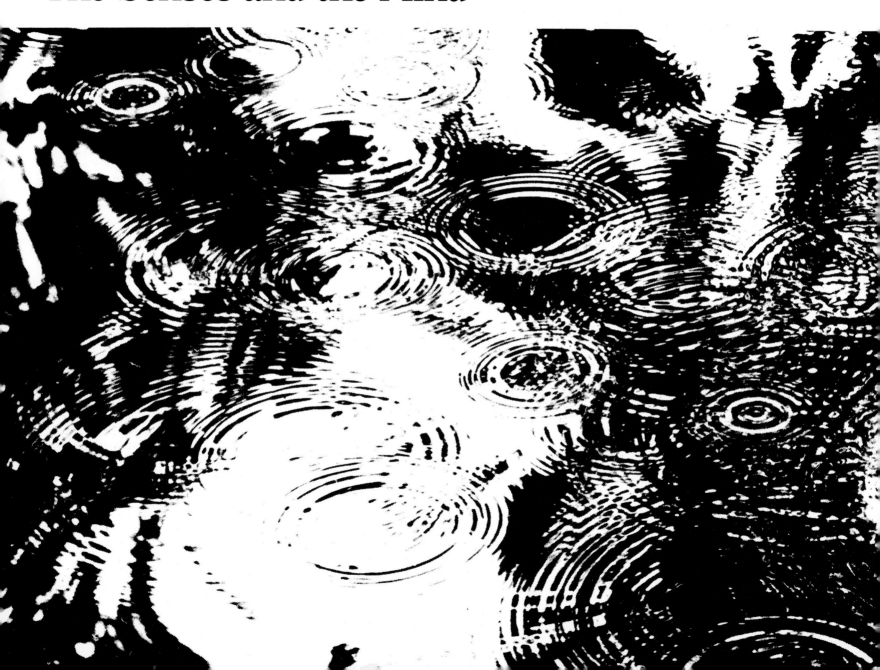

Chapter 9

How Can I Have a Relaxed Relationship to Influences?

The word *Pratyahara* means abstracting, leaving something, distancing or letting go. It has become a special yogic term describing the ancient method of withdrawing the mind.

You have now used the yoga exercises to prepare for the meditation. The body is not disturbing you any more and the breathing exercises have helped dissolve tensions. But despite your efforts, something else may hinder and disturb you. The idea of an ideal meditation and an ideal life can often be a barrier. In fact the attitude you have to life and to yourself can make the whole difference as to whether you lead a happy or an unhappy life.

Some people think that you have to live far out in the country to be able to meditate, while others furnish special rooms for the purpose and can't bear to be disturbed by family, neighbours, traffic...

From time to time, you may have considered moving into the country, but if you now, just now, don't live in the country or lack the possibility to withdraw, what do you do?

Many years ago, when I first heard about yoga and meditation, I was told how meditation is being able to live in the midst of life's bustle - and be yourself. Not buried in your own thoughts, but resting in yourself, acting freely from your own centre.

I heard about a man who had a well-run shop, a wife and a lot of screaming children, with the shop opening onto a street in the noisiest, busiest part of town. Yet that man could cut off at any time; wherever he was, he shut his eyes and entered a deep rest within himself. And when he reopened his eyes after any length of time, he was refreshed.

Pratyahara functions like this

Let us take an example of a smell:

The disturbance

I sit down about to meditate (or something else I planned to do; this method can be used at any time) and suddenly my nose is filled with a smell that won't go away. I don't like the smell, I call it unpleasant, it occupies my attention.

To become conscious

From my knowledge of this method, I start observing my nose and the smell there. How does it affect my nose? I experience this - it fills my nose and excites the olfactory organs. This affects my mind, which immediately judges it as unpleasant.

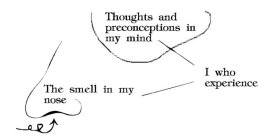

I surrender to the experience of the smell and saturate my mind with it ...

Instead of saying "ugh", reacting and suffering, I go into the experience and open my mind to it.

The experience becomes my meditation object. I see **the smell in itself**. I see the **thoughts** around it and I experience myself as **the one experiencing this**.

I realize that the smell and the thoughts are two different things existing each on their own. Therefore I can disregard the thoughts (abstract) and experience the smell, which is here anyway, no matter whether I am here or not, being disturbed by it.

I can also look at the thoughts as apart from the smell, and realize that they do not come from the smell, but from my habitual or instinctive reaction to such a smell.

In Pratyahara, you constantly observe the process of perceiving. That is all. You are consciousness, the one who experiences. You don't try to change anything, you just go on observing the smell and the reactions of the mind, as an alert, interested observer.

...and in that way the mind is satisfied and leaves the smell

That which the mind has experienced fully no longer interests the mind - this is its nature. The satisfied mind turns to something else...

The mind's interest in its surroundings is primarily focused on the conditions of your existence - on your needs and on what may threaten you. If you try to suppress a sound, smell or pain - a disturbance - you prevent the mind from studying it. Then the mind won't know if it is dangerous or useful. The mind, therefore, cannot let go and the disturbance remains (conscious or unconscious).

I had a student who told me that, to his astonishment, he had slept naturally for the first time in ages the very night after he learned step 1 of "Inner Silence" (page 99).

For years he had suffered from insomnia and, despite the experience, he couldn't really believe that just listening to the different sounds around him could have such an immediate effect. But I could give him an explanation:

"Years ago, you moved out of the city. But the city grew and moved with you. Now there are neighbours with children and dogs and traffic on the road has increased. You didn't like that, you let yourself become annoyed and in this way developed a negative attitude towards your irritating surroundings.

And now, for the first time in all these years, you experience it all as just sounds, not deliberately there to disturb you - the sounds are not hostile, they just exist, pure and simple - and this convinced your unconscious that no longer were there any threats around you. The result was that you dropped off to sleep safely and undisturbed."

The mind was satisfied and had withdrawn.

On this basis we can understand the ancient manuscripts. In the *Gheranda Samhita,* it says:

"Now I will tell you about Pratyahara, the best of all things. Mere knowledge of it destroys the enemies of man like greed, etc.

"Wherever the mind wanders, master it and lead it back.

"Do not let your mind attach itself to either praise or insult, master it and draw it back and hold it under your own influence.

"Bring your mind back if it goes to either a pleasant or an unpleasant smell. Keep it under your control by practising Pratyahara.

"If your mind is affected by sweet, sour, hot, cold or any other taste, draw it back with Pratyahara and hold it in your control."

In the *Yoga Sutras of Patanjali,* it says:

"Pratyahara is the withdrawal of the senses from their objects, in that the mind does not take the form of the object.

"Then follows the highest mastery over the senses."

But remember, you cannot use Pratyahara if you avoid both activity and trouble. Go on living as you do, meet life, meet problems - and in the midst of storms and stillness, experience... But how, you may ask. Is this expressed in concrete methods? Indeed it is.

When you are thrown off balance, first of all **accept** it, don't keep experiences at a distance, let them touch you. And experience...

At the end of this chapter we will take up some different methods but first turn to the Back Stretch and the Abdominal Stretch (pages 74 and 76) and see how you can relate to pain. Go through the exercises or use the method for whatever pain or tension you already have, then return to this text.

I want to tell you here about a student I had, a woman who suffered from asthma. She had very painful coughing seizures that she had suffered from for seven years.

One day I taught her the above exercises in class. At home she realized that this was not only useful in a yoga pose, but she could use it on the pain of her disease.

"I perceived," she said, "that I was at war with my own body. For seven years I had endured this hostility. I had nothing to lose, so I took a chance and began to accept the pains and allowed myself to locate and feel them."

For about three months she used this method constantly, and gradually the tensions disappeared and with them the pains. Then she removed the rest of the illness with the breathing exercises. When she told me this, there had been no trace of the disease for over a year.

She was one of my first students. Over the years many students have had positive results using this method.

In the Scandinavian Yoga and Meditation School we have weekly classes with yoga for pregnant women. It has become very popular to use yoga as a preparation for the birth. Not only the physical exercises and the breathing techniques, but also this method of Pratyahara.

One woman told me that she didn't want any sedation when giving birth: "I became so taken up by what happened, it was so exciting that I even forgot to use the special breathing

I had learned. When the pains sat in, and they really *hurt,* I chose to go into the pain and experience it. And then it all changed, the pain dissapeared, and I was fully concentrated inside the womb feeling the downward and forward movement..."

Many people tell me that Pratyahara is helpful with migrane and headaches. You locate the pain and hold on to it with a keen interest. In the case of migrane you may experience strong reactions from the body and you may also get lots of memories coming up. This can take several hours, but in the end you may even cure yourself of the migrane.

Just letting go and accepting the pain also works. A Finnish yogateacher suffered from articular rheumatism, especially in the hands. She had been with the school for several years, and although the yoga helped her, the disease still gave her a lot of pain. Then one day during a meditation, the pain disturbed her so much that she gave up the fight and surrendered to the pain. After the meditation she realised that this was the first time she had fully accepted the pain. During that same meditation the pain disappeared, and it never re-appeared to bother her again. This is now many years ago.

The main idea about pratyahara is that you withdraw from the influence. You can **decide** to drop the pain, just like that, it sometimes works. **Or** you can use this paradoxical method of satisfying the mind. If the pain is within a tolerable limit use it in the dentist's chair - I do that, and I find myself "forgetting" the pain.

People often ask me whether you run a risk of suppressing the pain and hiding a necessary symptom, or whether a healing actually takes place. In our society a very large number of people suffer from "psychic" pains. In Denmark, when the doctors can't help they often suggest that people try yoga. It is first of all such pains that is helped by Pratyahara, but not only. I believe that when you release a pain and relax the area, you also heal that area. After all, disease is most often caused by tension.

Don't get preoccupied with your sufferings, however, use pratyahara and forget them.

Little Yoga Nidra
Deep Relaxation

Now follows a relaxation, a Pratyahara technique in which you withdraw your senses, let go of stress and worries, and build up inner peace.

If you want to be guided into relaxation, use my tape *Experience Yoga Nidra* - two deep relaxations that will enrich your daily life.

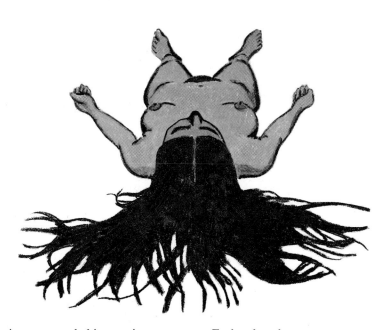

This text is written as a verbal instruction:

Begin by lying on your back with your hands at your sides and your feet a little apart. Cover yourself with a thin blanket. Lie completely still and feel your body's contact with the floor.

Feel how your arms touch the floor. Concentrate neither on your arms nor on the floor; imagine that you can feel the surface between them - between your shoulders and the floor, between your head and the floor;

the plane between your back and the floor, buttocks and the floor, thighs and the floor, calves and the floor, heels and the floor. Feel these points of contact. Under your heels, neither your heels nor the floor, but the space between them.

Stay with this a couple of minutes, then experience these points as one surface, one single plane of contact between them. Neither the body nor the floor, but the plane of contact in between. Feel the whole plane at once.

Feel a plane between your upper and lower lips.

Between your lips.

Feel your eyelids - where the eyelids touch.

Between your eyelids - between the lips - between the body and floor. Between the lips, between the body and the floor. Between eyelids, lips, body and floor. Between lips, eyelids, body and floor. Keep at this for a while.

Feel your whole body. No longer the plane of contact but the body itself. Experience the

whole body from head to toe. The whole body. It is lying as still as a tree-trunk. Experience the body as a tree-trunk. A motionless tree-trunk. Absolutely motionless.

But this tree-trunk is alive. Feel the body breathing. Notice air passing through your nose. Feel the air passing in and out of the nostrils.

Do not influence your breathing at all, but observe the natural breathing process. Natural breathing in and out of the nose. Concentrate on this for a while. Absolutely natural breathing.

Don't change it. Try not to give it any special speed. It takes care of itself, and you look at it.

Imagine that the air goes in through **one** nostril and out of the **other**, in the **other** and out of the **first**, alternate breathing in through one nostril and out of the other, in the other and out of the first. Always inhale through the nostril through which you have just exhaled. Go on with this.

In one nostril, out the other, in the other, out the first. Don't use your fingers, imagine it or feel it.

Then start counting. When you inhale through one nostril, say **one** (silently to yourself), out through the other, **one**; in through the other, **two**, out through the first, **two**; in through the first, **three**, out through the other, **three**; in through the other, **four**, out through the first, **four.**

When you come to **five**, inhale through both nostrils and exhale again through both.

Six, in through the first again; six, out through the other; seven, in through the other; seven, out through the first; eight, in through the first; eight, out through the other; nine, in through the other; nine, out through the first; ten, in through **both** nostrils; ten, out through both nostrils; eleven, in through one; eleven, out through the other.

Go on counting... and at 5, 10, 15, 20, 25, 30, 35, etc.: in through both nostrils, out through both. Otherwise alternate, in through one, out through the other, in through the other, out through the first.

Go on counting and see how far you can get

without making a mistake. If you forget to use both nostrils every fifth time, if you fall asleep or count incorrectly, start again. Begin again with one, as soon as you discover that you have made a mistake. But avoid making any mistakes, go as far as possible with the counting. Continue with this for some time. Exact counting, conscious counting and conscious breathing.

This exercise is also very good for insomnia: if you are lying awake unable to sleep, use this technique; and not only at night - if you use it during the day it will also improve you sleep at night.

Stop counting and feel your whole body again, feel it lying on the floor.

Imagine a blue sky and a bright sun, and that you're lying on a beach. Feel the warm sand. It's a lovely warm day, the sun's over-head, hear the sound of the surf, see the white sails out at sea, children playing on the shore, people bathing and lying relaxed in the sunshine, a warm summer day.

Feel your whole body, from head to toe. Feel your whole body.

Picture a mirror, think of a mirror, one you know well, see your own face in that mirror.

And now gradually come out. Become conscious of: "I am lying here on the floor". Start listening to your surroundings, gradually open your eyes, slowly sit up and look around the room.

Inner Silence
a Tantric Meditation

Step 1. To experience a totality
Settle down in a chair or in a meditation pose. Make sure your back remains straight, particularly the small of the back. It is important that you remain motionless and relaxed throughout the meditation. Close your eyes and come to rest.

This meditation is based on Pratyahara:

Start listening to your surroundings:
Listen in all directions.
Hear everything around you,
all sounds, in all directions.
Hear all the sounds around you
all at once, all the time, not just one sound
but all the sounds.
Consciousness is like a light,
shining in all directions,
shining on everything indiscriminately.
Consciousness perceives everything
with the same interest,
nothing is emphasized, nothing pushed aside,
notice a car in the street and a bird singing,
at the same time as the clock's ticking,
and as the neighbour's radio or TV is on.
Perceive everything around you, all sounds at once. 5-15 minutes.

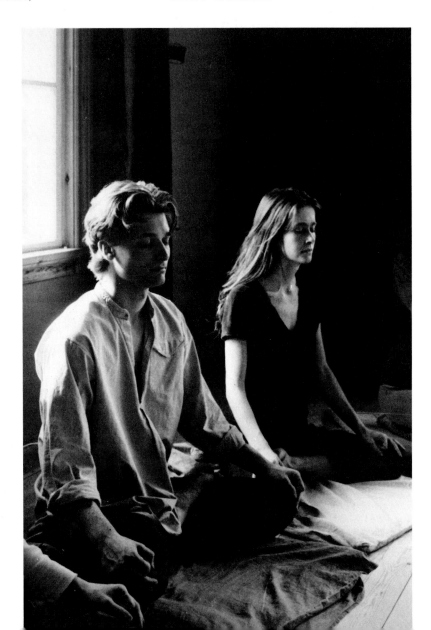

Do this once a day at home, also try it anywhere, any time, at work (take a minute to relax and experience yourself), in the bus (close your eyes for a minute), on the train, in nature or in the city.

Step 2. Spontaneous thinking

When you have experienced step 1 a few times, proceed to step 2. Put these two steps together, start with the sounds. When you feel that you are really there, at one with your surroundings as a whole, through the sounds, then allow your mind to turn to other experiences.

The mind is satisfied with experiencing the surroundings and it forgets to listen - see what makes it forget.
Be aware of whatever comes to your mind.
Let it wander wherever it wishes, freely.
Thoughts - emotions - moods - states.
The experience of your body,
well being, itching, pain.
Do not will yourself to experience anything specific, let your mind be free,
let it decide what to experience.
Relax completely and give yourself to this experience.
And while you sit this way, realize:
I am experiencing all this;
all around me, in my body and in my thoughts,
but behind it all, I am the one who experiences.
All is just experiences, which come and go.

You experience yourself looking at thoughts.
You remain yourself sitting, experiencing:
thoughts, emotions, preconceptions, opinions.
The observer - the silence on the background of which all activities are felt, seen and heard, that I am - alert and interested.

Do not analyse your thoughts,
do not be pleased or angry about them,
no, only experience that you are thinking, that is all.

Let each thought flow freely without restraint, no matter how provoking or tempting it may be,
the same with emotions.

I am the one who experiences the thoughts - the thinking process taking place in me.

What am I thinking right now?
- and now?
Now?

Go on, steadily and without interference, experience your own inner life -
let it happen, relax, accept it, experience.
I am not the one who thinks;
I am the one who sees the thoughts.

But sometimes you get carried away in thoughts and forget that you are meditating, and that's all right. When you discover it, look back at the thoughts again - consciously, and then go on.
The point is to experience
that you are thinking. How many or how few thoughts or emotions, or which ones, that is less important.
But to experience: I see that
the mind thinks - it thinks in me.
This is the essence of it all.

But remember that the instruction "I am not the thoughts, I am the one experiencing them" is not a weapon directed against your thoughts and feelings, it is not even a sentence that you repeat - it is your underlying attitude, the one that makes the meditation work in a liberating way.
And there are many ways of thinking;
you have your way and I have mine.
Perhaps you think in pictures,
perhaps in emotions, perhaps in words:
it is all the same.
Look at it - as an interested onlooker.
Notice when **worries** fill your mind.
What am I thinking of right now?
See the **opinions you have of yourself,**
see what dominates your mind

and decides for you,
consciously or unconsciously:
these thoughts I can think - these I suppress.
See the mind and all its contents
experience yourself as an observer.
Especially experience
the **spontaneous thoughts**
that appear by themselves,
apparently without cause,
just because they must surface.
See them as they are, brief fragments,
which normally, if you don't see them as such, turn into longer thought chains -
grow into broodings and memories
and make you forget yourself.

When you sit here you will learn
to contain all that you contain anyway.
And allow all contradictions to surface.
In this state you don't anxiously sort good (which you hang on to) from
bad (which you suppress)
but since everything is there anyway
you might as well admit it.
Experience it as an observer.
Let your mind go, let it drop its tensions.

There are no "good" thoughts
There are no "bad" thoughts.
Nothing need affect me
I let it all happen and just experience it.

But watch out that you don't become self-involved, that's not the point -
do not search for any thought or emotion, and **do not create any** -
experience only what comes by itself.
Let go and
stop letting the thoughts determine your life.
You are the one behind them,
they are just habitual patterns that you experience.

And yet dare let things influence you -
even let yourself get carried away
and experience the release of letting it happen and yet - deep down - observe it all with interest.

What did you think just now?
Look at the thought again.

Now and then you must allow yourself to be hit right in the heart - and see it.
It happens all the time, so instead of all those fruitless efforts to avoid it, relax, content yourself and experience what is happening anyway.

I am not these thoughts.
I am the resting-in-itself experiencing awareness.

Step 3. To think consciously and let the mind think

When you have worked at the first two steps for some time, when you can witness and let go of thoughts and feelings, then include this step in your daily meditation. Also return to page 10, "To transform inhibitions."

Experience -
First the sounds - then your free thought and emotional life.
After that proceed to choose one thought to think through,
one specific thought
or emotion that you know
you need to come to terms with.
Something you pushed aside,
something quite definite,
one subject, stick to it.
Think it through systematically,
stay with this one thought
or emotion. None of all the other thoughts can be present now.

Just this one subject - keep at it for a while and then abruptly stop.
For a while, hold the mind free of all thoughts. No thinking - no thinking.

Let the mind do it for you when you are in the state of meditation. Introduce a subject to the mind and let the mind do the rest. Here the mind has the capacity to think for itself. When you have chosen a subject for the mind to work with, watch how the mind treats the subject - don't interfere.
Give it a task or ask something, then look at it or listen to it and wait for the answer.

For instance, remember a recent walk, see again what you saw and did. Remember where the walk began and then let the mind tell you about the walk. Compare that to the way we normally try to control the mind. Do this for a while and find out the difference between the two ways of thinking - with or without the interference of your will.

This is a door to inspiration, when ideas are allowed to come by themselves; you don't look for them, they just appear, you don't have to make an effort or invent them. You ask your mind a question and the answer comes by itself. Or you consciously allow emotions that you would rather suppress to stay awhile, and then you finally dispose of them.

Re-experiencing through time...
Choose a specific theme: think back through today.

Just remember, go back through the whole day, the morning, the dreams before you woke up, last night, to the same time yesterday when you meditated.
Divide time into small units: experience here and now very intensely, and then go back one time unit at a time. (5 minutes or 15 minutes at a time.) Experience each unit individually. Do not leave out anything, not even "trivial" things - everything helps you to remember everything else.
When you have done this for a while you can also apply this method to earlier parts of your life, on any period of time that you want to re-experience.

...via places
If it is hard to remember periods long ago, then think of the places related to what you want to remember. I was in a house, then I was outside, then in another house, first in this room, then in that - you decide how to do it.

...via people
People you were together with - think about them and let the memories appear. Look at people from your past, let them begin to live and when that memory is exhausted, then think of someone you were with afterwards (or before).

... via an event
A third possibility: if you cannot get in touch with a specific place or person maybe you can remember something that took place at the time. And then that will trigger your memories of the people and the other things which happened.

...but avoid judging
One thing is very important in this context: do not judge what happened, just experience it - let it happen - re-experience it, but don't become attached to it.

Applications to dreams
Also use this method on your dreams - when you wake up, **lie completely still** and go back over your dreams.

Step 4. Let go of the thoughts

Now, as in step 2, your are the witness of your mind - but the moment you discover that you are engaged in a thought, you let go of that thought, you withdraw.
... if you like to feel one with your body (see chapter 11), then return to that, when you have left the thought.
... if you like to feel one with your breath, then return to that.
... if you like to feel one with your self (see chapter 12) then return to that. Be one with your self. And again, when you forget your self in a memory, in a plan or a longing, accept it, realize it and withdraw from it - back to your self - again and again. Be open for whatever new thought may surface. See the kaleidoscope of thoughts and emotions and remain your self experiencing them. Accept any experience, let it show itself, then drop it and return...

Part Four
Going Deeper

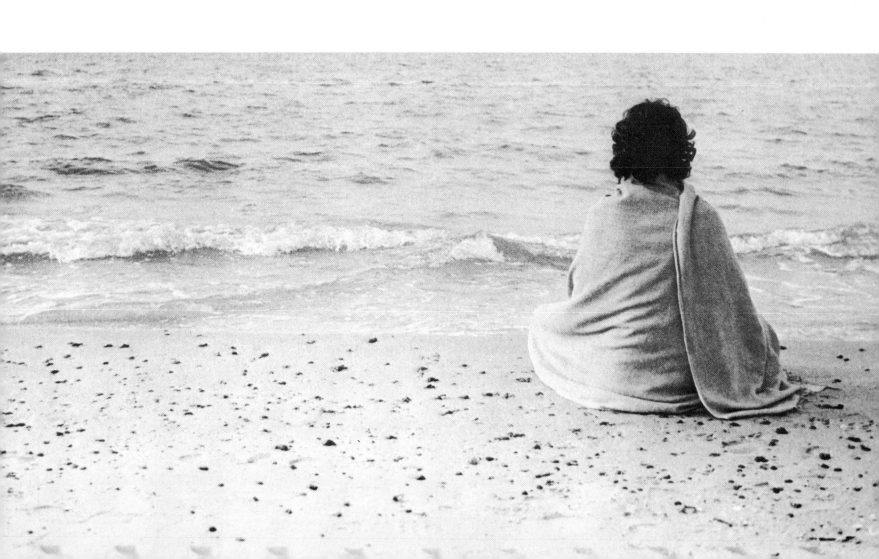

Chapter 10

Inspired Interest - On Concentration

Introduction

Meditation is a vast, many-faceted subject. In the three subsequent chapters I will treat it from different angles. And I will also discuss topics that apply to Inner Silence, the meditation described in the previous chapter.

One way to describe the path is by the following three steps to learning meditation:

The first step is called concentration: to be able to occupy the mind with one thing for a certain period of time; to be fully conscious of what you are doing all the time while you do it. Concentration is what this chapter is about, I call this step "inspired interest".

The next step is called meditation, meaning to be able to remain for a while in a relaxed and concentrated state. A state of "clear awareness", no matter what affects the senses or surfaces in the mind. That will be discussed in chapter 11.

The last step is a state of full consciousness.

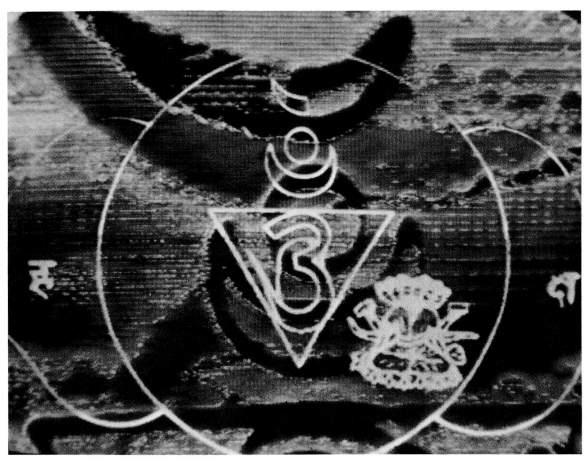

First you become one with the experience - or the meditation object - then you experience without being preoccupied by anything, inner or outer; you experience quite simply being yourself - as awareness resting in itself. See chapter 12.

There is also another thorough way, however, to describe these steps and I will do that here as an introduction to the following meditation techniques.

I would like you to think of concepts like coarse and fine. Take gravel or sand. Gravel consists of small and larger stones, coarse in comparison with fine sand on a beach that is constantly being washed and polished by the waves.

Sounds are the same, there are coarse and fine sounds. Think of something you shout out loud, something you say normally, words you whisper and those you think; shouting is coarser than thinking. Similarly, we can speak of coarse and fine vibrations e.g. sounds, light and radio waves.

In meditation the mind must have something to hold on to: a meditation object can be an image, idea or sound, which so occupies the mind that it enables you to get absorbed.

I distinguish between the three different kinds of objects as:

1. coarse
2. forms made of light
3. the very finest.

1. If you meditate on a candle flame, as described in one exercise in this chapter, obviously you'll be looking at a coarse object.

Many **coarse meditation objects** may be used. Strictly speaking, any image you see with the eyes could be used as a coarse object in meditation. However, the flame of the candle is very powerful as a concentrated radiating object. And it has a double effect, since you are also concentrating on the after image of the candle with closed eyes.

A daily practice with the candle over a period of time will enhance your capacity to visualize, and thus prepare you for the second step.

A meditation object is chosen with care, especially for the inner visualization of the second step. It must be something that appeals to you and holds your interest, something you can feel one with. A good meditation object works as a nucleus of power, as a centre of harmony, of light or of consciousness.

Therefore simple symbols are often the best objects. We find them passed on in Tantra, but we also find them in Nordic rock carvings, on Mexican sculptures, in Indian sand paintings, in Australian stone and cave paintings, which are painted even today, and they reach us from the ancient Egyptians. They are spirals, the so-called sun-cross, swastikas, crosses, an eye, a burning oil lamp, a burning candle, concentric circles, pictures of corridors, animal symbols, flowers opening, especially the rose and the lotus. There are symbols for the sun and the moon, and stars, also symbolically depicted as the pentagram: the five-pointed star; or the star of David: the six-pointed star. There is a crystal ball: as a symbol of the mind; an oval form or stone: as the symbol of the universe; the golden egg: as the symbol of life; and there are symbols like triangles, squares, circles or simply a dot. Or what you find in this book: the Tantric yantra.

I have mentioned symbols and yantra. There is a different meditation where you concentrate on one of the five elements: earth, water, fire, air and ether (space), or their corresponding sensory experiences: smell, taste, sight, touch, hearing and the experience of space. Or you concentrate on your own mirror image or shadow.

When experienced through the senses, these objects are coarse. In the first exercise: Tratak, intense concentration, you focus on such an object, the flame.

2. Take up the second step in the meditation, when the first Tratak, concentration on a coarse object, has been mastered.

This is called **meditation on the forms made of light**. Here the objects do not need any outer source of light. To perceive them we must close the eyes.

Images and symbols can appear when you do not anticipate or struggle. You just have to be **here**, fully aware. Obviously this is a finer form of concentration with great effect.

You choose **one** specific symbol either consciously or, better still, the symbol appears by itself during your meditation and it becomes your psychic symbol. This symbol you identify with and keep for life.

With the symbol you go deep in your consciousness, not hanging onto or being disturbed by anything inner or outer. The mind now has a point of reference and everything else, tempting or threatening, that appears in your consciousness is seen and allowed to pass by. I am the symbol. Thoughts, images, emotions or moods are something else. The symbol is all - you do not identify with the rest.

When I become conscious of the mind as such, I can avoid disturbing it or tensing in front of the experiences it contains. I can let it exhaust itself and relax.

We now have an effective method to release neuroses, depression and obsessive thoughts - and to make the mind creative, calm, full of inspiration and good ideas.

The *Inner Tratak* in this chapter will teach you to use this step. In chapter 11, I take it up in a slightly different way. The methods of this step are also used in contacting the chakras.

3. The third step is called **meditation on the very finest.**

There might be a difficulty here. **Talking** about this subject is very much a limitation, for it does not involve an **understanding** of words. When I suggest what to meditate upon in this step and you say, "I understand" or "I see", and then you think about it, that won't work! If you do that you find yourself back at

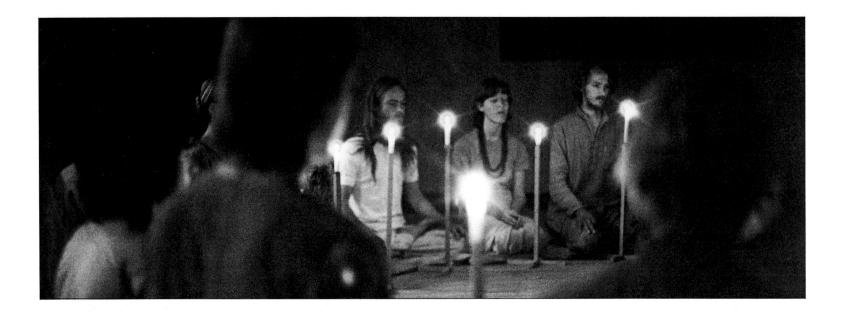

the beginning. The experience I describe has become a mere concept for your thoughts.

Do not begin this last step until you have practised the first two and have had results.

Let us look at a concept that we know well, especially from the art of painting. The abstract we will compare to the very finest. When, through the meditation process, we have left the different coarse objects, there will still be something left that we hold onto - that is abstract or fine in relation to everything else. A mind that is coarsely tuned will not be capable of perceiving this, because it thinks, judges, comments and calculates - in this step, however, we are dealing with **experience**. We do not tell ourselves what we do, see, feel or hear - we experience.

Therefore we must try this out, which we do in the exercise in chapter 12. Here I can only mention three examples, not to understand or describe, not to reflect upon, but to experience: *I - infinity - eternity*.

Tratak

Intense concentration

Tratak has many potential uses. The word can quite simply be translated as (intense) concentration. Tratak actually means unbroken gaze or attention on one object - to look upon or into.

The object need not be material, it can also be a visualization - an inner symbol or a chakra.

Tratak is a part of Hatha Yoga as a cleansing process and of Raja Yoga as a concentration method.

Through Tratak, you increase your ability to hold your mind on one thing, concentrated, as long as possible. This not only builds up concentration but also will-power and the ability to use your energy and yourself economically. (But the technique should be done in an easy, relaxed way.)

Tratak can be used as:

1. Therapy. Relaxation and eye exercise.

If you use Tratak as an eye exercise to strengthen your vision and to throw away your glasses, you would do it slightly differently from the description that appears later in this chapter. Certainly you use a candle, but instead of closing your eyes before tears come, you keep them open as long as you can without blinking, even when tears stream down your cheeks. But rest your eyes by closing them now and then. You may also find it more effective to look into the middle of the flame instead of at the glowing point at the top of the wick. To improve your eyes, you should do Tratak for five to fifteen minutes every day. I can recommend that you use other eye exercises together with Tratak (see page 63), as well as Neti, nose cleaning (see page 56).

2. Concentration. Tratak can be used to attain greater calm and concentration (for study and work) and to attain higher abilities, such as in *Prana Vidya* (knowledge of how the energy flows in the body), where you heal yourself and others by directing the psychic energy and by concentrating on tense and diseased areas (see also the previous chapter on Pratyahara).

By arresting the unconscious movements of the eyes, tensions are released in the brain. Tratak thus eliminates fatigue and results in natural, effortless concentration.

I have called this chapter **Inspired Interest**. With this kind of concentration, you need only to decide to do something and direct your attention to it; then in a natural way you will be absorbed in the work in question. The work becomes satisfying.

3. Meditation. Tratak is used for its own sake and as a preparation for more extensive techniques. Many other yoga and meditation exercises are enriched by the use of Tratak, as it makes the mind capable of visualizing, as well as receptive and sensitive to finer states.

Outer Tratak, Inner Tratak

There are two kinds of Tratak: outer (*Bahir Tratak*), gazing on an outer object or image with open eyes; and inner (*Antar Tratak*), "seeing", gazing or directing one's attention to an inner object without using ordinary sight, usually with closed eyes.

The first of the following exercises could be said to be a combination of Inner and Outer Tratak, but because the object we see afterwards with closed eyes is coarse, i.e. the candle flame imprinted on our retinas, it must be considered outer.

Inner Tratak is a separate meditation discussed at the end of this chapter.

After Tratak it is good to do the Little Yoga Nidra (chapter 9), then to meditate and merge with your personal symbol.

A couple of practical remarks before we start Outer Tratak: The room you sit in should be dark with the exception of the candle you use. If you wear glasses or contact lenses, remove them before you start.

Finally, and very basically: two seemingly

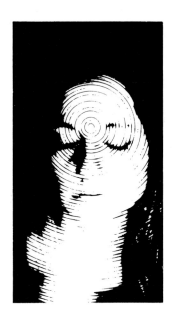

contradictory elements form part of the meditation. We could call them effort and relaxation; you either gather or disperse your field of attention; hold back or let go.

The two poles form the foundation for becoming conscious, for building up awareness. The whole work takes place between these two. When do you do one and when the other? It could easily lead to inner conflict, if you're not aware of the problem.

In Tratak you must be able to sit relaxed and do the whole exercise like a game, without straining - on the other hand you must stick to the exercise and do it precisely, without blinking or moving.

Don't overdo it. Do it at the most for fifteen to twenty minutes once a day.

Outer Tratak

Exercise:
Sit in front of a candle.
The flame is at eye level or slightly higher and 12 to 18 inches (30 to 40 cm) from your

eyes. Find the right distance for yourself.
Your back should be straight and your body motionless as long as you sit in this pose.
Feel your body as completely calm.
Experience the body's form
the whole body, for a while,
till you really feel it, until you are one with it.
The whole body.

Then observe the breath -
the natural breathing.
Observe the breath in your nose.
Feel how air goes in and out of your nose.
The natural breath in your nose.
Do it for a while.
The breathing in the nose.
When you feel calm, open your eyes
and look into the flame.
See the glowing point at the top of the wick.
Look at this point without blinking -
look as long as you can - without straining -
without blinking -
until tears come, or just before tears come.

When you feel a need to close your eyes,
do it, but don't move.
Sit completely calm and motionless,
with closed eyes
and look at what appears on your retina.

After a moment a light point is sure to appear.
This is the print of the flame on your retina.
You see a little star,
or a glowing point.
Look at it as long as you can.
Does it move?
Let it move to the centre between your eyebrows.
Look at it there.
If it wanders elsewhere, don't follow it.
Keep it at the eyebrow centre
as long as you can.

Sometimes the point vanishes,
then appears again
and then disappears.
And the point or background
may change colours,

the point may turn black
and the background light.
Go on looking at it until it disappears
altogether - it may take five minutes,
or longer.

When you are finished, stretch your body,
rest your legs if you need to.
And then settle down and start from the
beginning again.
Do this three or four times.

Meditation on the forms made of light.

Before you start with **Inner Tratak**, you must have thoroughly mastered Outer Tratak and become used to it. Only then is it recommended that this next technique be taken up. The most important rule with all kinds of meditation is **non-effort**.

A technique must be easy to do, it must be able to fascinate the mind and hold its interest.

Natural Concentration as a Basis for the Meditative State:

Before the actual state of meditation emerges, a state of concentration is experienced. This concentration cannot be associated with any form of effort or difficulty. It is something that happens all by itself as a result of the used yoga or meditation technique. You talk about the mind flowing into **one** point. All energy and interest is gathered automatically and effortlessly around one thing, one meditation object, gradually creating or triggering a state of meditation.

Now, it is quite clear that "nothing comes from nothing doing nothing". You must do something if you want to meditate; but if the technique appears more difficult than it appears attractive or effective, then there is something wrong with the way you use it. Maybe you have gone forward too fast or you have done too much. Maybe you have misunderstood something. Or quite simply you have the wrong attitude and make effort at places where instead you could rest in yourself and "follow" the technique in a relaxed way.

Strain during an exercise is often a beginner's problem, like sitting with tense eyes, especially when you have to use the inner sight. This is not at all necessary; Outer Tratak, yogic exercises and eye exercises are recommended to overcome these problems.

But in this context eye exercises are not enough. It is a question of learning to see the inner object at the eyebrow centre without thinking that you have to use your eyes.

Inner Tratak

This meditation instruction, which is transmitted verbally by a teacher to a student during the meditation itself, is long and detailed so that the student can keep alert all the time.

Exercise:
Adjust your body
and get ready for Inner Tratak.
Sit with a straight back without straining.
Be relaxed but keep your spine upright.
Eyes closed, hands on your knees.

Now slowly gather your attention
around the eyebrow centre.
Think of the centre between the eyebrows.
Feel the centre between the eyebrows
and see the centre between the eyebrows.

See it from within without straining your eyes.
See it instead from the brain.

It is very important in this technique
that you don't strain in the least.
If you feel you're straining,
then check yourself,
relax and give yourself to it.
Let this happen by itself.

See a little star, a little glowing point
at the centre between the eyebrows.

Experience this point
behind your eyebrow centre.
Experience it clearly,
it may suddenly appear very distinct
and then it may vanish.
That doesn't matter, go on, return to it again.
Or it may not appear,
it may not come at all.

Then think of a dark night.
The sky is covered with clouds,
a pitch black, dark night.
In the cloud, there is a little hole
and through that hole
one solitary star twinkles
out in the infinite universe.
Look at that star
experience that star
or think about it.
If you cannot feel the eyebrow centre,
put a little saliva on the tip of your ring finger
and place it on your eyebrow centre.
Make sure that the saliva is there.
Then take your finger off
and feel the saliva on your eyebrow centre.
Gradually, as it evaporates,
you will notice this area very clearly.
Hold on to this experience,
keep the eyebrow centre in your attention.

Then think about that time
you did Outer Tratak.
When you sat and looked at the candlelight.
After you looked at the flame,
you closed your eyes
and saw a spot appear on your retina.
Think about that point.
Think about that point,
that psychic point,
see it, a glowing spot.

What colour was it?
What colour is it now?
The spot you saw after you did Outer Tratak,
can you remember that spot?
Think about it, re-experience it,
see it at your eyebrow centre.
Now think about the flame.

Think about the candlelight that you saw
when you did Outer Tratak.
Let the image of the flame appear very clearly.
What did the candlestick look like?
And the candle, and the flame?
What did the wax look like?
What colour was it?
Was the flame white?
On the top of the candle where the wax melted,
and, where the black wick rose from the wax,
was the wick bent to the right or the left?
And the tip of the wick was glowing
and the flame surrounded the wick.
The flame was living, perhaps it flickered.
What colour was the flame further up?
What colour was it on top?
See the flame very clearly in front of you.
It flickers, it's alive, the wick burns.
On top of the wick is the glowing point;
the base of the wick is in melting wax
and further down the candle,
what colour was that?
And under the candle you had a candlestick.
Picture this in front of you.
What was the flame's aura like?
Can you see the halo around the flame?
What colour is it?
See the flame's radiance.
See the whole scene of the candle in front of
you and see yourself or experience yourself
sitting in front of the candle.

Once more:
Feel the centre between the eyebrows,
gather your entire attention around the centre
between your eyebrows,
hold your attention there.
Notice this place clearly
think about it, feel it and see it.
And if it helps, take a little saliva on
your ring finger and place it on the
eyebrow centre.
Keep your fingertip there a while so that you
are sure that it is wet. Then remove your
finger and concentrate on the spot.

If you can easily feel the place, then of course
you don't need to use your finger.

Hold your attention on the eyebrow centre
and see the little star there.
A shining spot, a little star.
See it clearly.
Or think of a dark, pitch black sky.
The sky is covered with clouds.
Think of a hole in the clouds
and see a little star twinkle
out in the infinite space of the universe.

And now remember the spot
that you saw when you closed your eyes
after looking at the candle flame,
the spot printed on your retina.
See that spot again.
Do you see it before you?
What colour is it?
Is it light or dark with a light background?

It doesn't matter what it looks like,
just hold onto the experience.
A little spot,
the reflection of the light on your retina.
If you cannot see this point,
then imagine a shining kernel of corn.
A little seed
A glowing seed.
See it clearly.
A little kernel
or just a glowing point, a shining point,
a psychic point behind your eyebrow centre.

Now see a human eye,
evoke the experience of a human eye.
A human eye with eyelashes, pupil and iris,
a complete human eye at the eyebrow centre
and you are looking into it
and it is looking into you.
See that eye,
distinctly experience the eye
at your eyebrow centre,
the image of a human eye.
Think of a human eye,
then experience it in your eyebrow centre.

Don't force it: if you strain, it won't work.
Let the eye appear of its own accord,
a human eye.

Now think:
behind the eyebrow centre
there is a little point,
and there is your psychic eye.

What we have been concerned with here
is your psychic sight.
You can see any image whatsoever,
gradually, as you become more trained.
This will strengthen your insight,
your thought capacity,
your ability to visualize and concentrate.

See the human eye again,
at the eyebrow centre.
And think of,
or move with your feeling
or with your inner sight,
to a point behind the eyebrow centre,
to a place in the middle of your head.
An eye is hidden there.
Picture that eye;
it is closed for the moment,
as if lips are closed around it,
but you know it's an eye,
you picture an eye like that there.
This is your psychic eye.
It is not open yet,
it's closed, but you can imagine it
or think about it.

Now see an oval form
standing on end.
Think of this oval form,
experience it, see it in your inner gaze.

If you are straining, it won't work at all,
just relax and think of an oval form.
See it very distinctly
this oval form.

And now see a clear, round, crystal ball.
Look into this absolutely clear ball.
Identify yourself with this ball -
become one with it.
Experience yourself.

OM TAT SAT - Inner Tratak is over.

Chapter 11

Clear Awareness - On Meditation

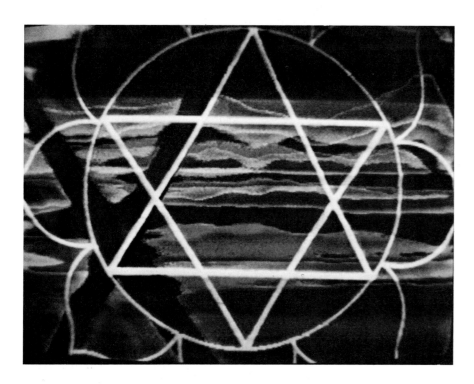

1. The transition from one step or state to another in meditation.

2. How mantra meditation according to the ancient tradition can be rediscovered.

Let us take a look at a party. The guests arrive. The party starts, gets going, more and more people loosen up and everyone has fun - the party reaches a peak.

Then it starts losing momentum, some people go home, and finally only a few exhausted people are left.

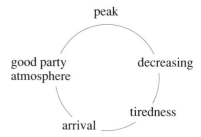

Those who left the party at its peak went home in a good mood and would probably wake up bright and fresh the next morning. You can imagine what it was like for the ones who kept on until the last...

We will later apply this example to the sequence of meditation.

The three basic elements in our meditation techniques are:

1. Body awareness

2. Breath awareness

3. Mantra - a syllable, word, or composition of syllables.

Here I will talk about the Tantric meditation sequence. You have already become familiar with the use of it in the two previous chapters.

The sequence is constructed as a step-by-step development leading from coarser to finer states. In the meditation you will use the coarse in the beginning as a warming-up and clarification process - which you must go through if you want to have a real experience of the final phase, the very finest, consciousness.

I conclude this chapter, with a technique in the Kriya Yoga tradition, a minor technique actually, but even so, one you will surely like. If you want to learn more about this kind of meditation and work with powerful methods, you must be instructed by a teacher who really knows them. Nothing compares with personal and direct transmission of the knowledge.

Before we turn to the exercise, let's discuss two subjects that will help you understand:

Body Awareness

To feel and experience your own body or its form is a fundamental and natural basis for meditation and relaxation. When you break your usual patterns of moving with yoga, or even in free movements and dance, you establish a new contact with your body. In yoga, awareness of the body has to do with moving, bending and stretching the body in different poses.

But to meditate on your body, as an immobile object that is filled from within with your awareness, till you become one with the whole body, is the foundation for one of the most profound methods: to perceive your own essence, your innermost being, "your actual form" - *Swarupa*.

Body awareness is in itself an experience and when you satisfy the mind with this experience, you go deeper. Through Pratyahara the mind loses interest in what it has experien- ced fully and turns inward. You have seen how this was applied to outer disturbances and pain and it also goes for the body as a whole.

The nature of the mind is such that it needs help to "go in"; it is not enough just to close your eyes. I have talked about different degrees of awareness: from coarse to fine. In the process of meditation you go from one state to another, you transcend. When the state has a lasting effect, it becomes a permanent transformation.

When you follow a technique, the state is changing by itself. You can't force a finer state even though it is more powerful than a coarse. In the beginning, you must follow a chosen and fundamental method. The mind will be satisfied and open to finer states.

So you start by practising body awareness.

Do it after your yoga and breathing exercises, and do it when you are tired and exhausted, after coming home from work or immediately after a long walk or jogging. In such a condition the mind will be inclined to let go.

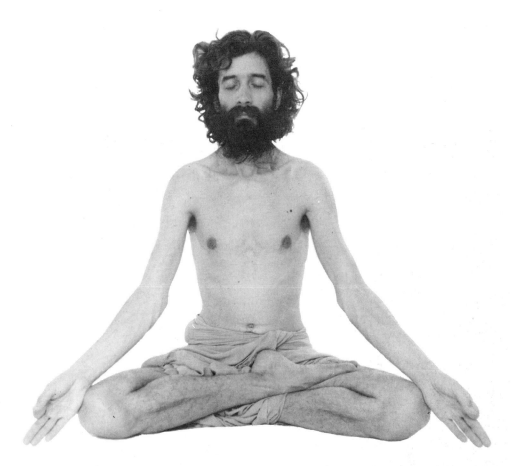

Also let go of any expectation, as it may block the real experience. When you repeat this exercise you get to know your body. You may have various experiences - but in the end, you will be experiencing yourself in your body: without thinking you will feel that you are one with it.

In this way, you attain a still greater unity between your consciousness and your body, and a still deeper concentration.

The change in your consciousness happens the moment you really feel one with the body. You may have the experience of sitting in a huge bubble of energy, or maybe you are filling the entire room... This is a temporary high point of the meditation - gradually you become familiar with it. Then you go deeper...

An exercise in Body Awareness

We have used this earlier in Breathing I and with Tratak, but here it is in a pure form. It can last from five minutes to one hour.

Sit in a steady pose - motionless.
Concentrate on motionlessness.
Hold this motionlessness
- nothing moves, your body mustn't sway -
not even your eyelids or lips should move.
Experience motionlessness.

This is the beginning;
go on for several minutes,
until the body really feels completely calm,
and doesn't need to move.

This is done relaxed.
Experience the body's relaxation:
your head is relaxed; brain, face,
chin and shoulders are without tension -
your back - and now - the whole body,
feel your whole body - relaxed,
the whole body at the same time.

Then think of
and feel the whole body as an object -
notice how it sits on the floor -
how it touches the floor.

Feel the whole body **at once** and see it
as if **from outside** sitting on the floor.
Then experience your body **from within**,

Check that your brain is relaxed,
that there are no tensions in your body at all.

Fill your body with consciousness,
feel everything from within
all at once - the whole body.

Become conscious of
I am in my body
I am my body
I am.

Experience your hands for a moment,
just your two hands, nothing else,
stay with your hands a while

and then again your whole body
the whole form of your body
the body's shape
experience your body's form
from within
from without
from within
become conscious of
I am my body
I am in my body
I am.

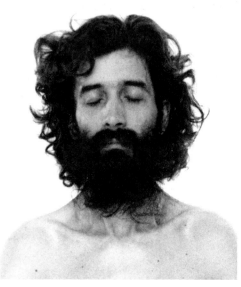

Breath Awareness

To be conscious about the natural or automatic breath is a meditation technique. In this context, it should not be viewed as a breathing exercise. You simply become aware of the breath which is always there in your body. You do not interfere with it. You experience that you breathe without obstructing, restraining, or accelerating the breath. It has its own speed and its own depth.

If you are breathless when you sit down - experience how it is to be breathless. The body is breathless for a while, then it calms down; let it happen at the body's own pace - by itself.

How is your breathing right now? Slow, dull, nervous or normal? Look at it without doing anything about it.

If you have difficulty in letting the body breathe by itself, do it lying down on your back; when you master this, do it in a chair or in a meditation pose.

Let the breath lead you from relaxation into meditation - to the experience of rest and being.

Let's see what happens on the way:

Firstly, the mind is trying to be involved with the breath, but you become sleepy - and it happens every time you have been sitting for a while...

You have reached the point in meditation where you have to cope with the threshold of sleep. And it may take some time before you get past this point (a week, a month, a year). Inevitably you fall asleep, or you get so tired that you give up meditating and go to lie down instead.

With the aid of an electroencephalograph (EEG) the nervous activity of the brain can be measured. The frequency we have shortly before falling asleep is the same as in the beginning of the meditation. When you have fallen asleep, the brain wave frequency changes, while when you meditate you keep the same frequency and the conscious state.

Without disturbing the body or tensing the brain, without getting out of the meditation, it is possible to keep awake within: give yourself time to observe this sleepiness - I am not this sleepiness, but I experience it - look at it as an object and **stay with it** as long as you can. When it disappears you will find yourself in a deeper and clearer state.

Secondly, the mind is trying to hold on to the experience of the breath, but all the time lots of thoughts pop up, continuous disturbances, brooding, impatience...

A tense brain is boring and empty of ideas: nothing really surfaces. The tensions hold your energy. When you practise breath awareness, the energy is moved from the inhibitions and they loosen up, the thoughts begin to flow more freely - the mind becomes talkative.

And you let it happen and become aware that you are experiencing it. You use the method learned in Inner Silence, step 2 (page 99) and the mind relaxes.

Some people say: "If I can't solve a problem, I just sit down and meditate and then the answer comes by itself." This has a simple explanation: a relaxed mind that you are not trying to force in a certain direction will sort out thoughts by itself. If you don't interfere the answer will come when the barriers and tensions are gone. A common example is when you can't remember a person's name and you say, "OK, I'll wait for a while and think of something else and it'll come to me." And that's right, that's how the mind works. Whereas, if you make too much effort, the mind will react by closing.

Thirdly, the mind tries to become one with the breath and it succeeds to such an extent that the breath becomes "independently alive" - it takes over your whole attention. There is nothing but breath, I am breath...

Thus the unconscious blocks of the breath are liberated, and you experience that the character of the breath is changing. It becomes deeply calm and rhythmic and at the same time it becomes lighter and in the end it almost feels as if you are not breathing. You are one with it.

You will not be able to force such an experience, it comes to you, and you follow it further and further... You devote yourself to the breath, without evaluating you relax profoundly and become one with the experience.

On page 43, you find the **practice** of Spontaneous Breathing.

Mantra

Runes of the mind thou shalt know if thou wilt be wiser than all other men.
                                    (from the Elder Edda)

In India personal use of a mantra is called *Japa Yoga*. There are numerous different mantras: *OM, Hum, Ram, Shyam, Klim,* etc. You get the mantra that fits your temperament and personality. It is important that whoever gives a mantra knows the effects of the mantras through his/her own experience in meditation.

A power or an experience is attached to the mantra initiation, and later this experience will come to you, when you have learned to use the mantra.

According to tradition you start by repeating (*Japa*) the mantra aloud (*Vaikhari*) a number of times. After you have been given the mantra and have used it for some time, your teacher should check it.

When you have warmed up and are sure of how to say it aloud, then you start saying it so low that it cannot be heard (*Upanshu*), but your lips are still moving. Each time you meditate you go through this process, repeating it until you feel you can go deeper. It comes of its own accord.

Let the mantra find its own rhythm or melody. This may be confirmed with the teacher and, if you need it, you should be given guidance concerning the experiences you have during the meditation.

In the third stage of Japa Yoga (*Manasika*), the mantra is repeated mentally and you experience how the mind becomes one with the rhythm or vibration of the sound. A variation is known under the name of Transcendental Meditation. Often TM is criticized because experience shows that many people at first get something out of using their mantra, but gradually feel that they are stuck in the same somewhat unreal state every time they sit and meditate. Eventually they tire of it and stop, since they don't get any help in going further in meditation. This, however, is not true of everyone.

When you express or think something, even if it is done very relaxed, then that action will create a counteraction - a reaction, and you must be aware of this in meditation.

In the fourth step of Japa Yoga (*Likhita Japa*), the mantra is written instead of said.

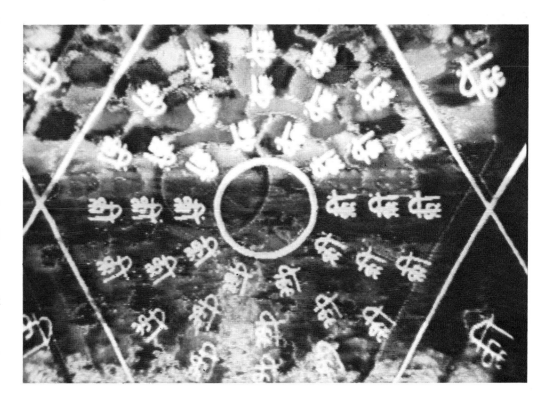

This means that you distance the "action" from your brain to your hand and thereby you also distance the reaction - all you do is experience your hand writing the mantra with red, blue, green or purple ink. The experience of the written mantra will influence your mind in a more gentle way than the previous stages. Sit still with your back straight and write the mantra as beautifully, slowly and minutely as possible - as many times as you can, it could well be several thousand times.

The final step in mantra meditation is often related to one specific mantra and one kind of breathing. This step is called "That which repeats itself without being repeated" (Ajapa Japa).

When you have experienced spontaneous breathing, you know what it means to let something just happen (the body breathes by itself). You let the breath live in itself and follow it, then "listen" to its rhythm and hear the Ajapa Japa mantra in it (see below).

You don't say the mantra; it appears on its own and you experience it.

In India the first three and the final steps are done with the help of a mala, a string of 108 beads on which you count the mantra. This way you become independent of time and don't concern yourself with counting the mantra; the mala and your hand do this for you, letting you become calmly absorbed in the meditation. And should you fall asleep, you drop the mala and that wakes you up.

You are now ready to understand the step-by-step structure and the aim of a meditation sequence. During the meditation, you go from one phase to another. To shed light on this I will construct such a course from the techniques just discussed.

You begin the meditation with the technique of body awareness. Follow it for a while, until you really get in touch with the experience of your body. At that point you will feel as if you transcend the body. Then at the peak of the experience, go to the next step.

Compare this to the description of the party at the beginning of the chapter - you reach a peak in body consciousness and just when it's at its very best, **without disturbing the experience of the body,** you let the experience of the natural breathing emerge and become dominating. You are now going deeper, and instead of experiencing a diminishing effect, you come in at the start of a new party, a still deeper peace.

And just as you become one with the breath and the breathing begins to have a deep effect, you start listening to the sound of the mantra in the breath. The breath fades away and the mantra becomes the most important... And you continue to add more subtle methods.

However, this is not based on superficial experiences. This kind of sequence takes from twenty to forty-five minutes and may be concluded with the meditation in chapter 12.

Ajapa Japa

Now we will go into a very precisely prescribed sequence based on the Ajapa Japa meditation. We reproduce it here in a simple version, *Vishuddhi Shuddhi* ; or *the Source of Energy*, as I call it. Ajapa Japa is divided into several phases, reaching from the coarser to the finer. You should practise them all when you sit down to meditate. The coarse parts are based on psychic breathing and on a mantra.

Start by sitting still in a meditation pose.

The Breathing

Psychic breathing is produced by a whispering, slightly hissing sound deep down in the throat, **not in the soft palate** but down near the vocal cords, like the sound made by a small child in a deep, relaxed sleep.

Concentrate on this sound in the throat and make it sound the same when you exhale and inhale.

A deep, calm, relaxed breath; breathe in with the sound and out with the sound in your throat. The mouth is closed. (If you are not sure how it should sound, contact a teacher who knows this breathing technique thoroughly.)

With this breathing you hold your tongue curled back, so that the tip touches the soft palate as far back as possible. But do not strain. This is called *Khechari Mudra*. It affects the relationship between mental activity (thoughts, etc.) and the physical body (breath, tensions, etc.). It also has an immediate practical effect; saliva production is stimulated so you avoid having a dry throat. In addition, it influences the nerves. Taoist Yoga asserts that the energy attained through meditation is lost if this mudra is not performed.

At first it may be awkward to hold the tongue in this position, **but only at first** (as when you learn to ride a bike). Keep at it and it soon becomes a habit.

Now you sit, breathing deeply, listening to the sound when you inhale and exhale. After a while - **without changing your breathing** - picture that each and every time you inhale you are charged with strength and energy. Each and every time you exhale, you let go completely and experience total relaxation. This part can be done as a separate meditation. Do it for a while before proceeding with the other parts of the technique.

The Psychic Passage and Air

Picture a channel, a psychic passage or current in the front part of the body between the navel and the throat.

1. As you inhale experience it as a flow of air moving upward in the passage from your navel to your throat.

2. Hold your breath a couple of seconds at your throat and feel the throat chakra, while you name it three times mentally: Vishuddhi, Vishuddhi, Vishuddhi.

3. Exhale and follow the air moving down to

the navel again. Feel for a moment the navel chakra and name it: Manipura, Manipura, Manipura.

Sit that way for a while and picture that air rises and falls in this psychic passage between the navel and throat, driven by the psychic breathing in your throat. Inhale, up; exhale, down. Continue this for 5 to 15 minutes.

4. Go to Vishuddhi on an inhalation, exhale and stay at the throat. With the next inhalation move with the air in a psychic passage that runs from Vishuddhi to a point in the middle of the top of the head. With the next exhalation descend again to the throat. Continue 5 to 15 minutes.

The sound in your throat continues throughout the following practice.

The Mantra

Now forget the "concept" of air or breath rising and falling and proceed to **hear** the mantra *So-Ham* in the sound of the psychic breathing. (If you have received a personal mantra which can be divided in two, you may use that.)

First use the mantra in the passage between the navel and the throat. When you inhale, **hear** *So* rise to your throat, then hold your breath naming: Vishuddhi, Vishuddhi, Vishuddhi. As you exhale, **hear** *Ham* flow down to your navel: Manipura, Manipura, Manipura. *So-Ham*, the mantra of the breath, relates to *OM*, *So-Ham = OM*.

Then use the passage in the head. First inhale and go up to the throat (Vishuddhi). Exhale and keep the awareness at the throat. With the next inhalation ascend with *So* from the throat to a point in the middle of the top of the head, pause there. *The Unknown Point* has no name. With the next exhalation descend with *Ham* to the throat. Up on *So,* down on *Ham.*

It is important to let it all happen by itself. Let the flow find its own way - let it show you for example where The Unknown Point is found.

Two passages, first the channel in the front part of your body, then the one from the throat to the point in the middle of the top of the head - now let them merge and move all the way from Manipura to the top of the head and down.

Go on with this for ten minutes to half an hour.

The Space

Remain completely motionless from now until the meditation is over. Stop the psychic breathing. Forget the passages and the mantra. Direct your attention to the eyebrow centre. Let it rest there until a certain intensity is reached, then let it slide back towards the middle of the head (with no strain, let it happen as in a dream). Here, from within your head, experience an inner space. Fill this space with consciousness.

You are in this space, you are this space.

Kriya Yoga

The above is the beginning of Ajapa Japa. The actual Ajapa Japa is a sequence based on nine phases. Similar breathing practices are used in a more powerful way, together with deeper-reaching meditations, that end with you being one with your symbol (page 22). It could have been described here, but that would have been unwise. It really should be learned from a teacher who knows its depth and all nine parts.

Following Ajapa Japa comes *Kriya Yoga,* a dynamic and at the same time profound tantric meditation. It contains more than twenty different *kriyas,* from strong physical and energizing processes to subtle ones that reach beyond the limits of the mind.

Kriya means process, and is a broader concept in yoga. The word is used about the cleansing processes: "Hatha Yoga Kriya", and about a certain state of mind and practice in

Raja Yoga. Even Ajapa Japa is sometimes called Kriya Yoga, but that should not be confused with the advanced tantric Kriya Yoga.

I experience Kriya Yoga as a powerful meditation giving a clearly felt increase of energy, a state in which it becomes difficult to hold on to tensions and depressions. It cleans out my subconscious mind in a more effective way than any other method I know. The strength that I generate makes it easier to tolerate and confront the content of my mind - my dreams become clearer. I am able to be aware of and accept that which would normally fascinate me or make me forget who I am.

Kriya Yoga is only revealed in the learning process. It is kept secret so that you do not block the actual experience with an intellectual understanding. And first you have to be properly prepared with meditations like Inner Silence (chapter 9) and Ajapa Jap.

The learning period lasts at least twenty-one days, preferable thirty-three days. During that time you remain silent - that is, not **one** word is spoken except by the teacher. As you don't have to express your opinion about anything, you do not so easily identify with old thinking habits. Therefore the stillness you experience increases your awareness. Your mind becomes calm and your receptivity finely tuned. You also don't make any notes: your memory should not be dependent on facts, nor on a piece of paper. Not just a little part of your brain, but your whole organism will be able to remember...

In Sanskrit, silence is *Mauna* and one who is always silent is called a *Muni.* Gandhi was silent once a week; it gave him peace of mind, and at the same time this very active man used the silence for his extensive correspondence.

But Kriya Yoga in itself is not silence. To be silent is only a part of learning it.

"Kriya Yoga converges all the energies, gross and subtle, into a point (bindu) in the middle of the mandala of one's being. This is the gateway to meditation ..."

(Swami Satyananda)

Chapter 12

Experience Yourself

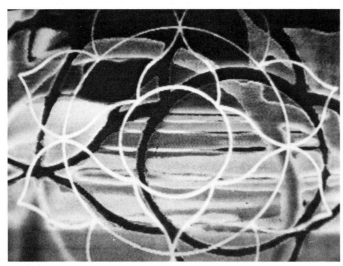

What is meant by Freedom and Consciousness?

Here I will not attempt to express an all-embracing truth, merely draw a perspective of the teachings of this book.

To be bound is to be the victim of inhibitions, tensions, compulsive thoughts and neuroses; the victim of fundamental forces such as fear, contempt, hate, desire.

To be free means first of all to be able to accept these forces and emotions; they are also part of me, I can learn to live with them or transform them. A strong method invoking this capacity you will have experienced in the Inner Silence meditation in chapter 9. And you have been presented with the idea of the psychic symbol as a point of reference in meditation. It helps you to distinguish the content of your mind and conquer the unconscious. "What you don't know, won't hurt you", the saying goes. However, this does not apply to tensions and unconscious

inhibitions - rather the opposite, "that which you can see, you can relate to and thus remain yourself".

When you are tired or depressed, when you feel tense without finding the cause, not seeing the inhibition you harbour - that you yourself have suppressed - then you are bound.

By becoming tolerant of the content of your mind, you will have the capacity to see more and more of that which influenced you unconsciously; it will then cease to disturb your peace or paralyse your vigour and self-expression.

Tantra is the method by which we can become aware of the unconscious forces - of what is there behind our emotions and thoughts, our states and energy.

Once you see through your expectations and see what is actually there, you allow the mind to accept what you see and experience it fully. But this does not mean that you analyse or "understand". When your mind is allowed

to experience, it becomes satisfied and loses interest, it relaxes and drops its involvement. It is no longer bound.

A tension or an inhibition expresses itself somewhere in the body or mind, somewhere in the different dimensions of your consciousness. But these dimensions do not include just tensions, they contain your life experiences, impressions and memories, your abilities and character traits. To describe how you let go of self-involvement in all these areas is to describe the process of becoming aware, a road to your real I - your self.

By steady concentration on one particular area you can see through and release the barriers, penetrate and go deeper, thus moving from plane to plane.

The mind turns from one dimension when it is satisfied by a complete experience and then it seeks something new to busy itself with - just as the mind in Inner Silence tires of sound and engages in thoughts instead.

Let us go through these different planes with the help of the methods we have learned.

We start outside, in our surroundings, the outer physical dimension, everything our senses can experience: sounds, smells... This was done in the first step of Inner Silence. For a while we stay with the sounds, remaining aware, until the mind is satisfied and turns to something else - and now we choose the body.

When you experience your body - your own physical dimension - completely, there will be a change. The mind will satisfy itself, and undisturbed by the body, the next dimension will unfold in your consciousness: the energy plane. Here you choose the breath as your starting point. By complete absorption in your natural breathing, you penetrate the energy plane and reach still deeper: to the thought dimensions.

You have your daily thoughts and cares, your plans and memories. When you have kept them for a while in your awareness, your mind loses interest in them and you go deeper. You may then meet the preconceptions that form your viewpoints. If you see through those, your frustrations, your hurt feelings or suppressed pride, whatever you normally identify with on an emotional level will show itself.

Rather than thinking "I am like that", you begin to experience yourself and from this viewpoint you see how your personality imagines itself: you experience the ideas you have about yourself... Actually you don't think that much when you meditate. You don't evaluate either. You just see and listen and experience how your consciousness has opened. With the help of earlier impressions, the mind creates the thoughts and images in which your personality mirrors itself.

Finally you can reach so deep in your meditation that the thoughts will be independent like dreams. Will they fascinate you and carry you away? Will you remain yourself, realizing that you are none of these deeply embedded influences? You are now reaching into the astral plane.

You don't think now, but experience things happening spontaneously. You can ask yourself a question before you start the meditation and your subconscious will come to perform a little drama as an answer or communicate through symbols. You even get answers or experiences without consciously asking. You may or may not get insight that way, but let these experiences pass by; don't destroy your meditation by evaluating what you see.

If you begin to take a position, discuss or explain your experiences to yourself, then you risk becoming involved again in tensions and deep-seated impressions. That which the subconscious tried to let go of will again be repressed by your prejudices or expectations and you will lose the clarity of your meditation.

If a tension clings, it will sooner or later influence your views, your breathing, your body and your environment.

In the state of meditation you don't become introverted or self-involved - you don't get lost in thoughts and images. You realize that you are the experiencing one. A thought is just an expression of an earlier impression, or perhaps a tension. When you let go of it, then harmony can have its way. Normally we attempt to exhaust these impressions through our dreams. The daily use of Inner Silence, of meditation, speeds up this process. Depressions, for instance, are seen and disappear because you don't identify yourself with them, they find nothing to cling to. You may be ill or depressed, or you may be exploring life, finding wisdom and energy - each time you go deeply into your mind, you may feel something spending its fury; you let it happen, and then you surface again fresher and stronger.

Let me tell you a personal experience of this:

A young woman who studied yoga with me came one day and asked to speak with me, saying she had a problem.

For a couple of weeks she had been obsessed by a thought and now it pained her so much that she had to talk to someone about it.

She had visited a woman friend and they were standing in the kitchen. A large kitchen knife lay on the table and suddenly the friend said: "Ugh, every time I see such a knife, I feel like grabbing it and sticking it into something or someone." "Well, that isn't very pleasant," said my student and attempted to give some advice. But when she left her friend, the obsession stuck with her. It was now three weeks and she still couldn't get rid of it. She asked me what to do, and I taught her a little about Inner Silence: next time that fear presented itself she should stay with it and allow herself to feel that obsession about knifes. However I did not ask her to behave in a "therapeutic" way, involving herself in worries and self-pity. As a witness, she should tolerate it, and at the same time exhaust it - watching her mind expressing the thought and letting go of it.

She would certainly do that, she said, and went home. That was in the morning. Towards evening, before I was to start the evening class, I was suddenly overwhelmed by tremendous fatigue. I sat down in a chair and

"went in" by focusing on my breathing - I wanted to relax - but suddenly there was a vivid, distinct image before my inner eye of an arm with a large, threatening knife.

My first reaction was, ugh, no, take it away! But just before I suppressed it, I was able to stop myself. I held on to the image - it was very vivid and now it started stabbing something. I kept the balance all the time so that I didn't suppress the experience but let it happen, held it there, while it got wilder and more alarming and at last it reached its bloody climax - then the knife began to move more slowly and the image rapidly became indistinct and finally disappeared completely.

I had suddenly become very alert and clear-headed. I felt full of energy and wanted to get going. My fatigue had completely disappeared even though scarcely five minutes had passed.

The thought of the knife never returned, neither to me nor to the two women.

But you are not yet near the cause, near the nucleus of tension, impressions and fundamental power. When you penetrate the astral plane (the subconscious) without identifying with it, you reach the causal plane

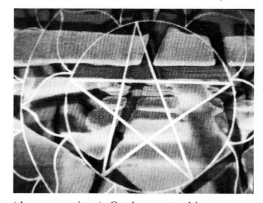

(the unconscious). On the way to this, we no longer experience sequences of events or dramas (dreams) but symbols, geometric forms, colour planes of many different dimensions. One profound, deep experience is, for example, that of a crystal universe.

Here experiences and impressions are "deposited" in the mind like crystals. The causal plane contains the essence of the impressions, the forces and deeper causes, rather than the single impression linked to a definite event and belonging to the dream plane.

Your psychic symbol can carry you through the unconscious and you start experiencing very intense light. If you get to this point, then you are **here** completely without any thought of body and personality.

And we've talked of other things along the way that could carry us there:

The name - *mantra* - took us part of the way, then the sound - *nada* - led us even deeper, and then with the symbol - *yantra* - we reached through the causal plane.

We passed through dimensions of different qualities and intensities, both coarse and fine; dimensions containing areas of varying frequencies - not only the physical or the mental, but the inner universe as well, experienced as light and sound vibrations.

We used the mantra and it became sound, we shut our ears and the sound became light, and the more totally we gave ourselves, the more our minds relaxed, the deeper and finer were the light and sound levels that came to us. Then, almost at the conclusion of the meditation we experience the bliss of being - *ananda*.

Meditation:

You will have to partly create this exercise yourself, including the order you do it in. I can only suggest a way to start or warm up.

Begin with the meditation you like best or else start like this:

I experience that I am sitting here.
Now.
I experience that my senses are directed outward to the world around me
except that my eyes are closed.

I hear everything around me,
I perceive my surroundings.
(Do this for a while.)

What is awareness in me?
Who am I?

I feel my whole body,
I fill it with my awareness -
my whole body at once,
its form, its fullness.
It is sitting here on the floor.
I feel it is still
I feel it is alive.
What experiences this?
What am I?

And breathing!
Do I impede it?
Do I quicken it?
Or can I let it
look after itself?
Can I experience it
interested but not interfering?
Who am I?
What am I?

Am I the thoughts?
Or do I experience them?
What preconceptions do I have
about all this - things,
the world around me, myself,
my personality, my name, my reputation?
What are my opinions?
These preconceptions come up in my mind,
tempting me to involve myself.
But I am not these.
I just let them pass by.
Who am I?

And emotions - I am not the emotions.
I don't seek them, I don't create them,
but when they come by themselves
I let them be, I even let them come to a peak.
I accept them
but I am not them.
I experience that I have them.
I am the one who experiences.

What am I?
Who am I?

Go on experiencing yourself
- not body, not thoughts, not emotions,
but you. Who are you?

And now experience contentment,
a contentment that fills you completely.
Evoke a deep inner joy,
not an artificial flight from something
but a state you allow to emerge
in yourself
from yourself.
I am sitting here resting in myself -
happy, deep inner joy
and contentment.
I -
Who am I?
What am I?

If you want
to make a decision
do it in this calm state,
in this deep rest.
Make a decision -
not a wish
but something that depends on your
self - something that you
in this deep peaceful rest in your self
decide
that you really want.

And go on now,
this is your own meditation.

Experience continuously
or again and again return
to the experience
Who am I?
(Don't ask with words any more,
don't answer any more - just
feel, experience.)
What am I?
I am...
all this.
Everything.

OM TAT SAT

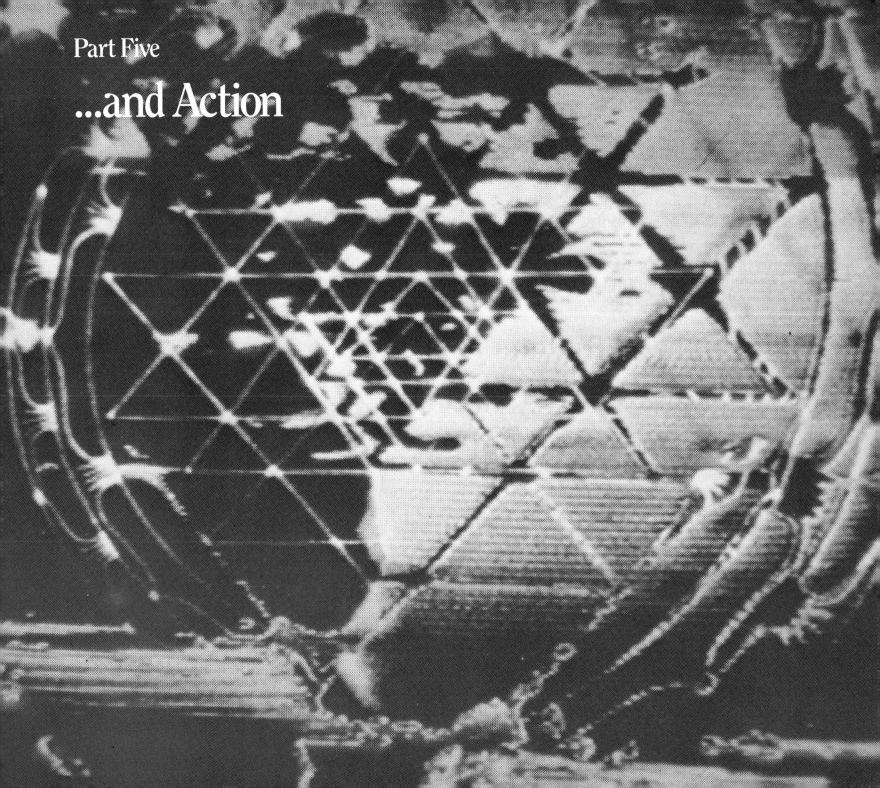

Part Five

...and Action

Chapter 13

Yoga for Daily Life

I'll begin this chapter with three dreams I once had.

"The Flight"
I had this dream many years ago when I lived in a little shop on a side street of Østerbro in Copenhagen. At the time I was living a very withdrawn life like an ascetic hermit.

I suddenly saw a huge wheel. It was made of human bodies, entwined together in ceaseless motion, like a whirlpool in a rapid torrent. And yet such a description is not sufficient, it was simply life, multicoloured and magnificent, overwhelmingly alive as it writhed in front of me. But down in one dark corner of this dream vision I saw a little bearded figure creep away from the wheel and leave the picture. This dream was stronger and more urgent than any I had had before; it was more like a vision, and it made me thoughtful.

Was I in the process of fleeing from life; was this a kind of self-involved suicide? Was I afraid to face difficulties or afraid of being beaten?

"The Director"
I had this second dream some years later, lying asleep one night under the starry sky in India, on one of the flat roof-tops in my guru's ashram.

I was still in a great "hurry" about my development - I did about five hours of yoga a day besides Karma Yoga all day long - but I was now very much more extrovert.

A while after I fell asleep, it seemed as if I awoke and looked up at the sky above me -

and there I saw a mass of people, a mighty stream of humans walking across the sky where I lay, thousands and millions pressing ceaselessly forward, all kinds of people. I saw many women and children in particular - and I saw a little figure rise up from where I was and start to get in contact with this mighty stream; it looked as if the figure wanted to direct the whole stream.

I had the third dream half a year before I finished my training in India.

"The White Robes"
I was standing wearing a white robe on a roof-top or rather on a tower, looking up at the heavens. The palms of my hands were joined at my chest as in prayer or greeting - I was totally absorbed in gazing into the sky. But suddenly something distracted me, something drew my attention away from heaven-gazing and I stole a look down at the street and there stood my guru beckoning me. I climbed down the tower and went out to the street to meet him. The street was an indefinite mixture of every possible country in the world. He looked at me searchingly and after a while he said, "Come here, you can handle more than that." He took me with him into the house and led me down through the vaults of the cellar, lower and lower, until we reached a large room with a great Indian well in the middle (such wells are 4 to 6 m. or 12 to 16 feet in diameter). He went over to the well, looked down into it and suggested that I go down - and I let myself be lowered into its depths.

And there are other dreams...

Behind much of yogic philosophy, behind much occult talk, behind much doomsday worship and sectarianism, there is often a desperate desire to be somewhere else, to get away as soon as possible to something other than the present. People talk of "the spiritual" and "the other side", but where are you in all this, where do you find peace?

What is here, is everywhere
what is not here, is nowhere

says Tantra.

From the way I have handled the subject of this book, it must be clear that I am not interested in starting a union of yoga practitioners, which would be as meaningless as starting a fellowship of toothbrushers.

No - but I like to communicate with each and every individual who wants to know something about working with him/herself. This work can take many forms and each of us must follow our own way - to ourselves. What that involves for you, only you can sense.

I aim to meet life as **my** life, as it comes to me, naked, without expectations which will be shattered by reality. Why dream your life away, why sit twiddling your thumbs, when there is enough to do right here, when there's plenty of life to live right now? Give up fear, says Tantra, and become one with life, as it is, hectic or calm. This is your own life, formed by you. And gradually, through work, through experience and mindfulness of your experiences, you achieve maturity that comes by itself. You don't have to wait - live.

Working with yourself can be compared to the work of the alchemist. For years he hammers at the same little lump of metal. He melts it down, then he hammers at it again for years. In the same way a tension, a way of thinking, has to be given up; the tension took root over a long period and a long time passed before you did anything about it, so - relax whenever you can.

When the tension returns - relax again. Keep doing it, no matter how many times it takes before it doesn't appear any more. With yoga and meditation, it goes as fast as it harmoniously can. But pay attention to your reactions - if you drive yourself too hard, your body and mind will react. Be quite clear about that, and let reactions come and go the way they do. Sometimes you won't be able to do anything - it seems like everything is afloat. Let it be, but be receptive when you feel like beginning again.

Problems are not removed just like that, but yoga gives you the strength to meet and experience them. You no longer need to be influenced by depression, you work with it instead. Do it indirectly by gaining energy from the exercises and directly by seeing the depression as an object. When you experience that you are looking at it, it no longer has any power over you.

Increased Sensitivity

As your senses and concentration are sharpened and your body gains strength, there is one thing that you must be aware of - you will be experiencing everything with an increased sensitivity, and life will be more a series of here-and-now experiences than ever before. What previously appeared to be difficulties now turn out to be experiences that are lived through.

You should know that not only all the tastes of everything you eat will be stronger but so will all the effects. A chocolate bar is not just a sweet; it will be a very powerful shot of (needless) energy, almost intoxicating, in the same way that tea, coffee and even herbal tea are.

I may eat a piece of chocolate occasionally, because I like it, and because it has an effect that I like to experience now and then. But just remember that if one day you don't understand your state, consider what you have eaten, what you have drunk: **everything** has an effect. The more sensitive you become, the more you see life this way: as a series of invitations that you can accept, but that you also gradually learn to take in the right quantity and use more consciously.

Clean Living?

When you take in artificial energy like sugar, tea, coffee or chocolate, the body's conversion of energy increases rapidly, and you'll notice it like a shot of strength. However, when the substance has been consumed, then the energy curve slides down below normal and you may get tired or depressed or else you crave another pick-me-up. To a certain extent, this is natural, but I have often experienced it as a disruption of the clarity that I achieve through the energy I have found in myself. This is not a summons to clean living (honey is, for example, to a sensitive person, stronger than tea, in that it gives intense dreams).

You don't have to be made over.
You become more yourself,
In the direction that you are going.

How much should you do?

Don't torture yourself, take a break now and

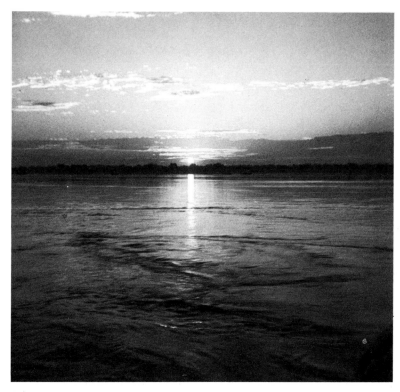

Sunrise

121

then. No one is making demands on you. Only your own desire will spur you on with the work. Do just enough of it; it should not be a burden. Make it expand your life.

It is good to do something regularly. Do a little programme with three to five poses, a breathing exercise followed by a little relaxation in the morning. In the afternoon after work, but **before** you eat, you might meditate for twenty to thirty minutes, for example using Ajapa Jap.

Time

Perhaps you want to do more: the morning is good for yoga and meditation, the late afternoon is good for meditation - and if you can't do yoga in the morning then it's fine in the afternoon too.

Before you go to bed you can also meditate or listen to the inner sounds - and this is also a good time if you want to do breathing exercises several times a day. Some maintain that you shouldn't meditate before you go to bed, because then it will be hard to fall asleep. If you suffer from insomnia, do the Little Yoga Nidra in which you count breaths in your nose before you intend to sleep (see page 98).

In my personal experience, meditation (and even yoga) in the evening brings nothing but calm sleep with clear dreams and lucidity in the morning.

You are your own authority. To have something explained and justified is only a hidden form of a need for authority. Try out the different methods and observe their effects - in that way you get a greater freedom.

Perhaps you are striving for a high goal, and you believe that you have to make a real effort in all that you do. But yoga doesn't work that way. Clenching your teeth will make you overshoot your goal. Do it all without expecting results - soft and relaxed. If possible do yoga regularly and avoid switching from periods when you suddenly do a lot to periods when you do little if any. That will not create stability.

If you have taken a break - no matter how short or long - let no conflict or conscience prevent you from beginning again when you feel like it. After all, to suddenly feel like doing something one day does not mean that you are obliged to carry on forever.

Yoga for Daily Life...

Above all, listen to yourself. How much can you manage, how much do you want to do, how much do you need? You're not doing these things for their sake, after all, you're doing them for your **own** sake. You could hardly call it a hobby! It is more a natural way to get in contact with yourself, and a simple, hygienic process - like washing, sleeping or brushing your teeth.

Thousands of books have been written about yoga, meditation and similar subjects. If you have read more than five, then maybe you should not have this one, especially if you don't feel like using what is in it. You won't get anything at all from reading it if you haven't decided to use it and do the exercises and meditations described.

Everyday life is not techniques or exercises, everyday life is reality - and reality may be easier to handle using yoga and meditation.

...and Spontaneous Meditation

Periods with intensive meditation and yoga such as holiday and weekend courses remind you of who you really are: existence, consciousness - and happiness (you don't worry). Later on, in the middle of your normal activities, you will be able to spontaneously recall and rely upon this experience. When you feel like it or need to be yourself, now and then, listen to this need and close your eyes for a few minutes.

You can - when you feel isolated or strange - acknowledge and live through the experience overwhelming you, and let it express itself in your body and mind, exhausting itself. And then you can return to the joy of the company of others.

You can shut your eyes for a short time, finding yourself. When you have high ideals about meditating and cannot stand the demand of doing extensive meditation at regular hours, you can, just for a while, listen to the sounds - people talking, traffic, machines, birds - and briefly experience your breathing (with or without *So-Ham*), then the inner space, and the symbol or yourself - and for thirty seconds experience yourself. Then open your eyes and go on with whatever you were doing before.

Going Deeper and Unfolding

Yoga and meditation have an effect. Therefore it is important to find the right balance between becoming absorbed and expressing yourself.

To give yourself and be active in life with the awareness you get through yoga is the way out of introversion and self-indulgence. Do something for others for instance. Whatever you do, do it as precisely and as well as possible. Don't leave anything for others that you could do just as well. Thus you will sharpen your powers of observation and achieve a greater perspective; and in meditation you avoid losing yourself in dreams and illusions and you will be able to go really deep.

The more you unfold and the more actively you participate in normal life, the more you will be able to meditate. If you are an individual who doesn't want to achieve anything and wants to relax all the time instead, then you might as well stop meditating.

Break out of your self-involvement, turn yourself outward. A yogi is a person who does not worry about how he or she feels - the goal is deeper, the perspective greater.

Take up different tasks without being too concerned about results. Whatever it is, do it as well as you can, and if you fail at something, start again. What makes you happy is not the result but the fact that you did your best. So get going again!

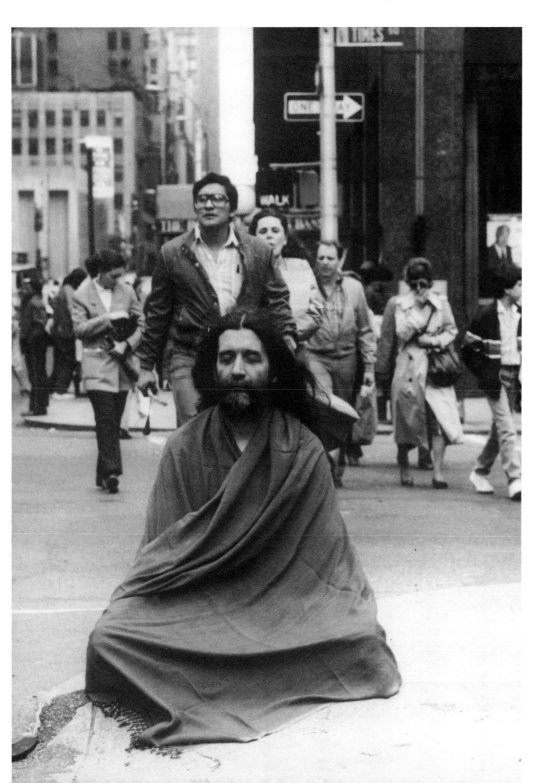

Toil and trouble...
(friendly) was it difficult?
(relaxed) oh no.

You can calmly
take pleasure in
what you're doing
right now.

No doubt
it will
change into something else
that you can delight in
when the time comes.

OM TAT SAT

123

Index and Glossary

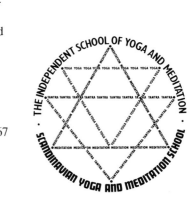

If you want tapes or further information on yoga and meditation methods and courses in Sweden and around the world, please contact:

Scandinavian Yoga and
Meditation School
S-340 13 Hamneda
Sweden
Phone: +46 372 55063